LEARNING
TO BE
HEALTHY

The Wider Benefits of Learning Papers

1 *Modelling and Measuring the Wider Benefits of Learning: A synthesis*
Tom Schuller, John Bynner, Andy Green, Louisa Blackwell,
Cathie Hammond, John Preston and Martin Gough

2 *Evaluating the Benefits of Lifelong Learning: A framework*
Ian Plewis and John Preston

The Centre for Research on the Wider Benefits of Learning
Institute of Education
20 Bedford Way
London WC1H 0AL
020 7612 6900
website: *http://www.learningbenefits.net*
email: *info@learningbenefits.net*

The Centre for Research on the Wider Benefits of Learning is an independent research centre funded by the Department for Education and Skills. The views expressed in this work are those of the author and do not necessarily reflect the views of the Department for Education and Skills. All errors and omissions remain those of the author.

LEARNING TO BE HEALTHY

Cathie Hammond

Centre for Research on the Wider Benefits of Learning

Institute of Education | Birkbeck College

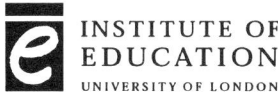

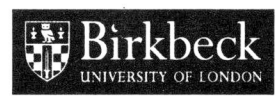

First published in 2002 by the Institute of Education,
University of London, 20 Bedford Way, London WC1H 0AL

100 years of excellence in education

British Library Cataloguing in Publication Data
A catalogue record for this publication is available from the
British Library

ISBN 0 85473 661 1

Cover and text design by Tim McPhee
Page make-up by Cambridge Photosetting Services, Cambridge
Production services by Book Production Consultants plc,
Cambridge
Printed by Watkiss Studios, Biggleswade

Contents

Preface

The Green Paper entitled *The Learning Age* (1998) sets out the government's vision for learning:

> Our vision of the Learning Age is about more than employment. The development of a culture of learning will help to build a united society, assist in the creation of personal independence, and encourage our creativity and innovation.
>
> (paragraph 8)

To take forward this vision, the DfES has funded a number of research centres to provide a stronger research base for the development and implementation of policy. The first of these centres to be established, in 1999, was the Centre for Research on the Wider Benefits of Learning (WBL), based at the Institute of Education. It is looking at the links between learning and a number of areas. One of these is health; the others are active ageing, civic engagement, families and parenting, and crime.

Compared to the extensive bodies of work on factors affecting participation in learning, and on the economic effects of education, there has been little investigation of the outcomes of learning that are not primarily economic. In part this is because of inherent difficulties in data-gathering, but perhaps it is also because the 'benefits' of education have been assumed to be obvious. One of our tasks is to probe more deeply into these relationships, and to develop better models for examining them.

This is the third paper in the WBL Centre's series. It derives from the first phase of the Centre's work, which involved reviews of the links between learning and functioning in the domains listed above. Further studies of the relationships between learning and family functioning, and learning and social cohesion are nearing completion.

Health can be both a cause and a consequence of learning. In this book, we focus upon one side of the relationship – health as a consequence of learning, and the processes through which learning impacts upon health.

John Bynner, Director of the Centre for Longitudinal Studies,
Institute of Education

Acknowledgements

I would like to acknowledge the support and advice of the following: John Bynner, Leon Feinstein, Martin Gough, Lars Malmberg, Deborah Safron and Tom Schuller.

Chapter 1

Introduction

BACKGROUND

Over recent decades, the body of evidence on health inequalities in Britain has been growing (see for example Marmot *et al.*, 1984; Black *et al.*, 1982; Acheson, 1998). That is to say, it has become clear that health status differs across demographic categories of the population, such as those defined by social class, gender and education. In response, major programmes have been launched by the Department for Education and Skills (DfES) and the Department of Health (DoH) which strive to improve health at individual and community levels through community regeneration, involving educational interventions.

One example is the recent establishment, during 1998 and 1999, of 26 Health Action Zones (HAZs) in England in areas of deprivation and poor health to tackle health inequalities through local innovation. HAZs comprise partnerships between the National Health Service, local authorities, the voluntary and private sectors, and community groups. They represent a new approach to public health because they explicitly link health to regeneration, employment, housing, and, more significantly in this context, to education. Education is used not only to raise awareness and levels of motivation but also to build self-efficacy and social cohesion. For example, projects involving education funded by just one of the HAZs in London include training in the use of the internet for older people in order to prevent isolation, Mental Health Partnership Conferences, Citizen's Jurors (which are like mini focus groups), action research projects, training of members of linguistic minority groups in health advocacy, as well as more traditional forms of health promotion.

Health Improvement Projects are similar to HAZs but operate on a smaller scale. Recently (in 2000) introduced in England, they set out the strategic framework within each Health Authority for improving health and reducing inequalities. Included within these frameworks are policies linking education and training with health.

An initiative that has been funded jointly by the DoH and the DfES is the National Healthy School Standard (NHSS). The NHSS recognises the potential of schools as settings where the health of children can be improved and comprises an infrastructure linking Local Education Authorities with Health Authorities, the provision of advice, training, and support materials, and a process for accreditation. The NHSS emphasises a 'whole school approach'. In other words, health promotion is achieved through the provision of information and guidance within an inclusive school ethos that develops amongst all members of the school community a sense of belonging, self-esteem and self-efficacy. Initial evaluations indicate that schools that have adopted the NHSS do, indeed, have positive effects upon the health of their pupils.

These initiatives result from developments in the understanding of the psychological and social causes of health and ill-health. Health is promoted not only through raised awareness and self-efficacy, but also through social cohesion. Education and learning are integral to each part of this process. In other words, they are seen as instrumental in developing awareness, self-efficacy, and social cohesion. These potential roles of learning are reflected in the government's Green Paper, *The Learning Age*, quoted in the preface, which presents a vision of learning as a means to build a united society, create personal independence, and encourage creativity and innovation.

This is the context for the following review of evidence about the processes through which learning affects health.

WHAT DO WE MEAN BY EDUCATION AND LEARNING?

Up to this point, the terms learning and education have been used without any distinction being made between them. However, they do not mean the same thing. All education involves learning, but learning is much broader than education. Most authors agree on the following distinctions.

Learning is a psychological process that can take place in any context. In contrast, education is more socially and culturally bound, usually taking place in institutions. Whereas education incorporates a prescribed curriculum and thereby intention, this is not a necessary part of learning. Both processes involve activity, whether this is in the form of creating the stimulus-response pathways of behavioural psychologists such as Pavlov and Skinner, the generation of new insights described by cognitive psychologists such as Kohl, or the development of cognitive maps (Tolman). In the literature reviewed here, most of the research draws upon learning in an educational context. The most common measures used are years of formal education and levels of qualifications gained, which probably relate more closely to education than learning, but which do not measure either concept accurately.

Years of education and highest level of qualification fail to capture the heterogeneity of education in terms of learning experiences (content of learning, learning styles, student mix) or learning context (type of college, type of school). This inevitably limits the conclusions that can be drawn from the review.

LITERATURE FROM WHICH THE REVIEW IS DRAWN

The mechanisms through which learning affects health cut across traditional academic disciplines. The relevant evidence can be found in the bodies of literature that relate to education, economics of education, economics of health, medical sociology, health education, health promotion, health psychology, and medicine. To cover all these areas in depth is beyond the scope of this review and so the emphasis has been to provide an overview based upon material published more recently. The econometrics literature will be addressed in the future work of the Centre.

Findings from studies conducted outside Britain are included, although the historical, cultural, and other contextual factors that influence relationships between education and health differ between countries. Therefore, findings from other countries do not map directly onto British experiences. Nevertheless, where similar effects are found, they may reflect universal patterns in the relationships between education and health. Where they are not, the disparities may inform our understanding of factors that influence these effects.

SUMMARY OF FINDINGS

The evidence for positive correlations between years of education and health status relating to physical and depressive conditions is robust. However, this on its own tells us nothing about causality. Health could be a cause or a consequence of learning. This paper focuses on the evidence relating to one direction of causality; namely, how learning affects health.

An obvious way in which learning has an impact upon health is through its effect on people's economic conditions and social status, and there is considerable evidence for the significance of this mechanism. In addition, an individual's education can affect access to and uptake of medical services. Other studies of the effects of education upon health have focused upon health-related behaviours. It appears that education affects health behaviours both through shaping attitudes and by enabling individuals to behave in accordance with them.

Outcomes of learning include improvements in self-esteem, self-efficacy, inter-personal trust, anti-discriminatory attitudes, access to a wider social support system, and social and political engagement and activity. These outcomes are instrumental not only in changing health-related behaviours, but also in increasing resilience – the ability to cope with adverse conditions and stress-inducing circumstances. Individuals who are more resilient experience lower levels of chronic stress in response to a given set of adverse conditions or stress-inducing circumstances. Living with high levels of chronic stress has adverse affects upon health, and so it follows that greater resilience will be beneficial to health.

Learning has an additional role in improving health at national and community levels through building social capital and social cohesion, and through reducing material inequalities. All these are associated with better health outcomes at community levels.

In this study of learning and health the following themes emerge:

- The immediate psychosocial outcomes of learning are of central importance in generating behaviours, skills and personal attributes that have early but lasting effects upon mental health, and cumulative effects upon physical health. This is illustrated in a model of the mechanisms through which learning affects health in Figure 1.
- The effects of educational experiences upon health vary depending upon characteristics of the learner, the learning context, and the learning experience. This has policy implications for decisions about investment in the types of learning that generate those psychosocial outcomes of learning that are particularly effective in improving psychological, mental, and physical health.
- Reducing inequalities in education may be more effective in improving health at national levels than providing more education for all.

The next chapter presents evidence for correlations between learning and health, followed by a consideration of the different models of causalities that may explain the correlation. Chapter 3, which is the core of the book, focuses upon one facet of possible causality, namely learning affecting health, and discusses possible mechanisms through which learning makes us healthy. The conclusions of the review are presented in Chapter 4.

Chapter 2

Correlations and Directions of Causality

CORRELATIONS BETWEEN EDUCATION AND HEALTH

The measures of learning and health used in empirical studies limit the scope of this review. As noted above, the most common measures used for learning are years of formal education and highest qualification attained. Measures using qualification levels exclude all learning that does not lead to accreditation, whilst years of formal education do not include attendance at evening classes, short periods of education and training, learning through work and non-work experiences, watching television, and discussions with family and friends, which fall within the parameters of learning as described in *The Learning Age* (paragraph 8). Moreover, these measures do not capture the focus, depth, teaching styles, or any other aspects of the learning experience or learning context.

Health status, like experience of learning, is also difficult to measure. Measures typically include mortality rates and morbidity rates for specific conditions, although some studies include self-reported ratings of general health and malaise. Most self-reported ratings are well validated. For details of the validation of self-rated general health status, see for example Power and Bartley (1993: 135).

Bearing these caveats in mind, the evidence for a correlation between learning, as measured by years of education and highest level of qualification, and physical health has been well reviewed (e.g. Ross and Mirowsky, 1999; Grossman and Kaestner, 1997). The overwhelming conclusion is that the evidence for a correlation is robust:

> A number of studies in the United States suggest that years of formal schooling completed is the most important correlate of good health.
> (Grossman and Kaestner, 1997: 73)

The correlation has been found worldwide and amongst individuals of different ethnic groups, ages and incomes. Some of the evidence is summarised in Tables 1 and 2.

Apart from physical health, there is also consistent evidence that education, as measured by years of formal education and qualification level, is correlated with happiness and lower rates of depression. The more educated individuals are the less likely they are to commit suicide. Details of some relevant studies are summarised in Table 3.

The results from recent surveys in the British cohort studies show that associations between qualification levels and health outcomes are not only statistically significant, but also substantial in magnitude. Data from the British cohort born in 1970 (BCS70) show that respondents with no qualifications were, at age 26, almost four times as likely to report poor general health as those with the highest educational qualifications (23 per cent compared to 6 per cent: Whitty et al., 1998). Analyses of the most recent sweep of the comparable cohort born in 1958 (data are taken from the National Child Development Study or NCDS) also report a substantial gradient in self-reported general health across educational level, with 35 per cent of 41-year-olds with highest educational qualifications reporting good health as compared to only 17 per cent of 41-year-olds with no qualifications (Feinstein, 2001). In relation to depression, the magnitudes of associations are also substantial. Parsons and Bynner (1998) analysed data from the 1996 sweep of the NCDS and report that 36 per cent of women and 18 per cent of men who had very low literacy skills suffered from depression, compared to 7 per cent of women and 6 per cent of men with good literacy skills. The relationships were smaller but still very substantial in relation to numeracy. Eighteen per cent of women and 11 per cent of men with very poor numeracy skills suffered from depression, compared to just 5 per cent of men and women with good numeracy skills. The magnitudes of these associations may be underestimates because Mackenbach *et al.* (1996) find that those who have completed fewer years of education tend to under-report illness.

In addition to the associations between an individual's learning and the same individual's health, there is an extensive literature that explores the connections between parental education and infant and child health. Much of the relevant research here has been funded by the World Bank and relates to developing countries (e.g. Glewwe, 1997; World Bank, 1994). Here, associations between maternal education and child health are found, but the nature of the education, which is often aimed towards health promotion, and the economically, socially, and culturally determined causes of infant morbidity and mortality are so different from those in developed countries that it is difficult to make comparisons.

Studies based in the USA conclude that the education of parents, particularly mothers, is associated with the health of their children, as measured using neonatal and infant mortality rates and rates of low birth-weight. For example, Corman and Grossman (1985) report that during the 1970s, neonatal mortality rates in the USA were correlated with whether or not mothers had at least a high school education, even after controlling for perinatal and neonatal care and maternal poverty. The death rates for infants with mothers who had not attended high school as compared to the death rates of infants with mothers who had attended high school was on average 1.7 percentage points lower for white families and 1.3 percentage points lower for black families. Between 1964 and 1977, increases in levels of maternal education accounted for a drop in the death rate of infants during the first month of life of 0.7 per thousand for black families and 0.5 per thousand for white families.

Grossman and Joyce (1990) report findings that, in New York City in 1984, mothers with more years of formal education had higher birthweight babies, even after controlling for age, marital status, health-related behaviours, type of birth, and antenatal care.

However, correlations between education and health are not always found, and when they are, they are not always positive. For example, the evidence relating to the connections between education and anxiety disorders is inconsistent. Beekman *et al.* (1998) report a correlation between level of education (low, middle, or high) and *lower* rates of anxiety disorders in young and old people in Amsterdam and evidence from an Icelandic study suggests that a correlation exists between more years of education and *lower* rates of phobias amongst older people (Arnarson *et al.*, 1998). On the other hand, Benham and Benham (1982) report findings that suggest that those with more years of education tend to suffer neuroses *more* than those with fewer years, and the evidence for a correlation between having higher levels of education and increased risk of eating disorders is consistent (e.g., Westermeyer and Specker, 1999; Toro *et al.*, 1995).

In a study of well-being, Veenhoven (1996) reports strong correlations between individuals' level of education and their happiness in poor nations, but weak and even negative correlations in wealthier nations. More recently, Wottiez and Theuwes have analysed data from a national survey of Dutch residents aged 43 to 63 and found no evidence for a correlation between years of education and well-being (1998). Veenhoven suggests that a possible explanation for the weakness of correlations in rich nations is the lack of high-level jobs.

Numerous studies of the epidemiology of chronic fatigue syndrome/myalgic encephalomyelitis (or CFS/ME) – in contrast to chronic fatigue – suggest that prevalence rates are particularly high amongst individuals who are of higher socio-economic status, which correlates with years of education and qualification level. Similarly, Heinrich *et al.* (1998) report that atopic disorders (i.e., allergies) are most frequently diagnosed in children of parents with higher qualifications.

It is important to investigate these variations in the correlations between education and health because they potentially provide clues about the nature of the connections between education and health and why they exist. Consequently, they are particularly relevant to Chapter 3, where I discuss mechanisms through which learning affects health.

DIRECTIONS OF CAUSALITY CONNECTING LEARNING AND HEALTH

The observed positive correlations between education and health can be explained in three ways. First, individuals with better health may be more likely to continue in education for longer and obtain higher qualifications. Second, one or more factors, for example family structure, income or parental levels of education may affect both education and health outcomes. These first two explanations are often referred to as *selection bias hypotheses*. In other words, individuals select to continue and/or succeed in education on the basis of characteristics such as family background variables and early health status, which themselves predict health status later in life. The third explanation, which is sometimes referred to as *social causation*, is that increases in education result in improvements in health. These three explanations are illustrated in Figure 2.

The evidence (some of which is presented below) suggests that selection bias hypotheses and social causation hypotheses contribute to observed correlations between education and health. This implies extremely complex patterns of inter-relationships that will change throughout the life course.

Health effects upon learning

Gilleskie and Harrison (1998) suggest that better health status enables one to achieve a higher level of educational qualifications (p. 280). It is also plausible that poor physical and mental health constitute barriers to successful learning and education. Evidence that physical and mental health affect educational attainment is presented by Edwards and Grossman, 1979; Shakotko *et al.*, 1981; Perri, 1984; Wolfe, 1985; Chaikind and Corman, 1991; and Wittchen *et al.*, 1998 and 1999.

Researchers have attempted to identify the causalities underlying the widely recognised association between the onset and progression of schizophrenia (and related psychotic disorders) and socio-economic status. Compared to their healthier counterparts, individuals with a diagnosis of schizophrenia or psychosis tend to have lower socio-economic status – often measured by years of education or highest qualification attained. This could be because individuals of lower socio-economic status are predisposed to the development of schizophrenia – the social causation hypothesis. An additional explanation (since the two explanations are not mutually exclusive) is that people with a diagnosis of schizophrenia tend to drop in socio-economic level – they do not enrol on or complete courses of study, they take employment of lower status or become unemployed. This explanation is referred to as the 'drift hypothesis', and it is an example of a selection bias hypothesis.

A review of the evidence relating to each explanation concludes that the one that accounts most convincingly for the association between schizophrenia and psychoses and socio-economic status is the drift hypothesis (Hare, 1983).

Factors that affect both learning and health

The second explanation for the correlation is that one or more factors determine both educational engagement and success, and health (e.g., Rosenweig and Schultz, 1981; Fuchs 1982). General material conditions such as housing and income levels clearly affect both people's ability to achieve in education and their health levels. But we have more specific information in some respects, namely in relation to income inequalities, future orientation, and cognitive and social functioning.

Wilkinson (1996) has examined the relationships between financial inequalities, educational standards, and health in Britain during the 1980s. Using data referring to income inequalities from the Central Statistical Office, data relating to the reading standards of 7-year-olds collected from Local Education Authorities (LEAs) (plus data from one LEA relating to children's performances in mathematics), and mortality rates in England and Wales, he demonstrated that during the latter 1980s, financial inequalities increased, educational standards dropped, and decreasing mortality rates slowed in very similar ways. Although the patterns in the data do not demonstrate causality, on the basis of theoretical and contextual argument Wilkinson suggested that growing financial inequalities resulted in simultaneous deteriorations in education and health at national levels.

Fuchs (1982) has suggested that persons who think within a longer time-scale, or whose thinking is more future-oriented, both attend school for longer periods and make greater investments in their health. Grossman and Kaestner (1997) refer to this suggestion as the time preference hypothesis, and cite studies that suggest that it has relevance to the observed association between education and health (e.g. Farrell and Fuchs, 1982).

It also appears that levels of cognitive and social functioning affect both educational achievement and mental health. Low intellectual ability indicated by an IQ measure below 90, and poor psychological functioning may be determinants of poor mental health (Kjelsberg, 1999; Jiang *et al.*, 1999, respectively). Impaired cognitive functioning during childhood is associated with an increased risk of developing schizophrenia and depression in later life (Bergman and Walker, 1995; Toppelberg and Shapiro, 2000). British and Swedish studies indicate that young people who develop psychotic disorders as adults tend to be poorly adjusted socially during childhood and adolescence (Cannon *et al.*, 1997; Malmberg *et al.*, 1998). It is likely that young people with poor social adjustment find education in institutional contexts difficult, and also that intellectual ability and cognitive functioning affect the level of education attained.

Learning effects upon health

The third explanation for the correlations between learning and health is that learning brings about improvements in health.

The hypothesis that learning causes changes in health can be tested through the quantitative analysis of longitudinal datasets. The best measures of learning available in these datasets are years of education and highest qualification; however these are more accurate measures of education than of learning. Because data are available about the histories of individuals, it is possible to investigate the relationships between education and subsequent health status, controlling for health status before school age, and before any other educational interventions. In addition, it is possible to control for background variables such as family income that could affect both success in education and health. However, even with longitudinal datasets, one can never entirely rule out the possibility that variables not included in the analysis account for part of an association.

For example, using two British national longitudinal datasets (the National Child Development Study (NCDS) and the 1970 British cohort Study (BCS70)), Bynner and Egerton (2001) performed regression analyses and report correlations between highest qualification gained and health outcomes at ages 33 (NCDS) and 26 (BCS70). The measures for health include risk of depression, self-rated general health and risk of assault and accidents. The correlation persists even when background characteristics such as maternal education, maternal interest in child's schooling, father's occupation, family income, housing, and cognitive skills at age 11 are controlled for. The implication of their findings is that something about qualification level has a positive *effect* upon health.

Magnitudes of associations between education and health tend to be overestimates of the effects of education on health, especially where childhood health is not controlled for, as it is not in these analyses. Bearing this caveat in mind, for the cohort born in 1958, respondents with degrees and above were about 1¾ times more likely to report excellent health at the age of 33 than respondents with qualifications below A-level. Amongst the younger cohort, born in 1970, and rating their health status at age 26, the difference across qualification level was not so great, with those with degrees and above about 1⅓ times as likely to report themselves in excellent health as those with qualifications below A-level. This is partly because the range in health outcomes is narrower at age 26 than at age 33. In relation to depression, having a degree as opposed to qualifications below A-level reduced the chances of becoming depressed at age 33 by about one-third for women and just over a half for men.

Recent analyses of data from the 1999 sweeps of the NCDS and BCS70 show smaller associations between qualification level and health outcomes, but use a statistical technique (propensity score matching) that is more effective in terms of establishing causal links. Variables that are controlled include childhood physical and mental health, childhood ability, attributes and attitudes, as well as family background variables (Feinstein, 2001). One possible reason why Bynner and Egerton find effects of education upon health that are larger in magnitude than those found by Feinstein is that they include more selection bias effects, as well as the effects of education upon health. If this is the case, then Feinstein's figures will be the more accurate estimates of the sizes of effects of education upon health.

An important finding of Feinstein's analyses, found also by Bynner and Egerton, is that the relationships between qualification level and health outcomes, especially depression, change depending upon the level of education, i.e., these relationships are non-linear. This raises important and policy relevant questions about which aspects of education are important in terms of improving health status across different groups of learners. Further research is needed to address these issues. However, some possible explanations are those discussed on pp. 26–7. Here, for purposes of comparison with the findings reported from Bynner and Egerton's analyses above, I report the effects of having a degree or higher level of qualification as compared to no qualifications. Also reported are some of Feinstein's other findings that illustrate the non-linearity of the relationship between qualification level and health outcomes.

Feinstein reports that for the 1970 cohort, the estimated effect of having a degree or higher level of qualification as compared to having no qualifications is an increase in the probability of reporting good health of 6 percentage points for men and 11 percentage points for women. He also finds effects in relation to respiratory problems for those born in 1958, with graduate men 17 percentage points less likely to report respiratory problems than men with no qualifications. The difference is statistically insignificant for women, but substantial nevertheless (11 percentage points).

Differences in rates of depression between those with a degree or higher level of qualification and those with no qualifications are not statistically significant except amongst men born in the 1970 cohort (whose chances of developing depression drops by 8 percentage points if they have higher qualifications), once all confounding variables have been controlled for. The only effects that are statistically significant across both cohorts are Level 2 qualifications (i.e. between O-level and A-level) as compared to no qualifi- cations for men and women, and for women only, Level 1 qualifications (below O-level) as compared to no qualifications. Having Level 2 qualifica- tions as compared to none reduces the probability of having had an episode of depression at age 33 for the 1958 cohort by about 4 percentage points for men, and by 5 percentage points for women, and for the 1970 cohort at age 26 by about 3 percentage points for men and 6 percentage points for women. For women, having Level 1 qualifications as compared to none reduces the probability of experiencing depression rather more substantially, by 7 percentage points for the 1958 cohort and by 11 percentage points for the 1970 cohort. These findings have clear implications about the importance of making education at a basic level accessible to those with no qualifications.

The picture in relation to training is very different. Highest levels of training appear to have significant protective effects as compared to no training for men and women in both cohorts. Perhaps this is because training is associ- ated more tightly than education with success in employment and integration into the workforce.

Models in which education is assumed to have a causative effect upon health have been tested in numerous other studies based upon data from other countries. As mentioned above (pp. 3–4), contextual factors that may influence relationships between education and health differ between coun- tries, and so findings based upon data from the USA, Nicaragua, Denmark, and so on will not map directly onto British experience.

Grossman (1975) estimated the schooling effect upon self-rated health amongst a sample of white middle-aged American men who had all graduated from high school. Controlling for health in high school, parents' education, physical and mental functioning when the men were in their 20s, current hourly wage rates, property income, and job satisfaction, he found that education had a significant and large causal impact on self-rated health. Using econometric models to analyse data from a survey of low-income men living in the USA in 1974, Desai (1987) found significant positive impacts of years of education completed upon self-rated health and significant negative impacts of days of work lost through ill-health. The results control for numbers of chronic health conditions (as a measure of underlying healthiness), the use of preventive care, and overcrowded housing.

Wagstaff (1986) estimated a health model based upon data from the 1976 Danish Welfare Survey using maximum likelihood methods. He found that more years spent in education leads to better health outcomes. Behrman and Wolfe (1989) estimated random and fixed effect models and concluded that for women in Nicaragua, years spent in education positively affected their health, even after controlling for ability, knowledge and tastes.

To conclude, reviews of the relevant evidence agree that the evidence for a causal effect of education upon health across different countries is consistent and convincing (Grossman and Kaestner, 1997; Hartog and Oosterbeek, 1998; Ross and Mirowsky, 1999). For example:

> Educational attainment has positive effects on health. The well educated experience better health than do the poorly educated, as indicated by high levels of perceived health and physical functioning and low levels of morbidity, mortality, and disability'.
>
> (Ross and Mirowsky, 1999: 445)

There is evidence that all three directions of causality described in this chapter together account for the observed correlations between education and health. This will generate feedback loops, whereby educational success generates healthier outcomes, which in turn predispose the individual to further educational success, and vice versa. Additional variables affecting both health outcomes and educational engagement and success will feed into these loops, possibly to differing degrees over the life course. Consequently, overall explanations for associations between education and health involving all three directions of causality are likely to be extremely complex, and the job of disentangling a single strand of causality is not a straightforward one.

The following chapter focuses upon just one of these strands of causality: the effects of learning upon health.

Chapter 3

Mechanisms Through Which Learning Affects Health

The inter-relationships between learning, health, and other variables throughout the life course are enormously complex. In their 'Input Paper' to the Acheson Report (Acheson, 1998), Whitty and colleagues refer to 'the cumulative effects of low social class of origin, poor educational achievement, reduced employment prospects, low levels of psychosocial well-being [upon] poor physical and mental health' (Whitty, *et al.*, 1998: 642). The task of unravelling such a tangled pattern may seem overwhelming, but with the rigorous application of statistical techniques coupled with qualitative analyses, it is possible to make headway in identifying independent mechanisms through which education affects health. Their independent identification does not, incidentally, imply that each mechanism operates independently of the others.

Whitty *et al.* suggest that 'education has both a potentiating and a protective role – potentiating in relation to the triggering of healthier lifestyles and behaviour, protective in that higher levels of education provide access to the kinds of employment opportunities and life chances that can protect individuals from disadvantages in later life' (1998: 643). In the same paper, they examine the roles of social capital in relation to effects of education upon health. In addition, The Ottawa Charter for Health Promotion, developed in 1986 as part of the World Health Organisation's strategy for health promotion, stresses the centrality of power and control in health promotion (Kickbusch, 1990). The importance of personal control is recognised by Mirowsky and Ross in their research investigating relationships between education and health (Mirowsky and Ross, 1998; Ross and Mirowsky, 1999).

In this chapter, I discuss five groups of mediators through which learning affects health: economic factors, health-related behaviours, resilience, access to medical services, and healthy societies.

ECONOMIC FACTORS

Probably the most obvious mechanism through which learning may affect health is via economic factors. Findings of a study based upon a large-scale survey in the USA suggests that about half of the effect of education upon physical functioning amongst adults over 60 is mediated by economic factors such as income and work conditions (Ross and Mirowsky, 1999).

There is strong evidence that educational success is associated with higher earnings, reflecting both higher occupational status and lower rates of unemployment. For example, Johnes (1993) uses findings from a number of authors to examine relationships between years of education and earnings and shows that investment in education is associated with higher earnings in both developed and less developed countries. In the UK, he demonstrates positive economic returns to education both for the individual and for society in relation to secondary and higher education, and across a wide range of subject areas. A recent literature review of the economic returns to education in Europe, edited by Asplund and Pereira (1999), concludes that education is associated with an increase in earnings that more than compensates for the investment costs of additional years of schooling (for at least some years) in all the fifteen countries studied. Chevalier *et al.* (1999) survey the available literature on returns to education in the UK and present some new estimates of returns using a variety of specifications and nationally representative cross-sectional and longitudinal datasets. They suggest that returns to education are lower for men than for women and that they rose over the 1980s and have been fairly static since then, at approximately 7–10 per cent for men and 8–12 per cent for women. These figures mean that for every additional year spent in formal education, earnings averaged over the lifetime increase by 7–10 per cent for men and 8–12 per cent for women. For further discussion of relationships between education and economic outcomes, see also Becker, 1993; Joseph Rowntree Foundation, 1995; Esping-Anderson, 1993; Psacharopoulos, 1994; Sloggett and Joshi, 1998; and Bynner and Roberts, 1991.

Higher earnings, higher socio-economic status and lower rates of unemployment are associated with better physical and mental health. The Whitehall study, which began in 1967, shows a steep inverse relationship between the employment grades of civil servants and their morbidity and mortality from a range of diseases (Marmot et al., 1984; Marmot et al., 1991; Hemingway et al., 2000). A government-commissioned report, entitled 'Inequalities in Health' and referred to as the Black Report after its author, published in 1982, demonstrates that the findings of the Whitehall study are not peculiar to civil servants and presents evidence for a clear gradient across socio-economic status running throughout the UK from those who are both socio-economically advantaged and relatively healthy at one extreme to those who are socio-economically disadvantaged and relatively unhealthy at the other. The more recently commissioned Acheson report, published in 1998, presents similar findings and suggests that 'the range of factors influencing inequalities in health extends far beyond the remit of the Department of Health' (Acheson 1998: v). For further reading on this topic, see Wilkinson, 1996; National Health Strategy, 1992; Nolan, 1990; Kunst and Mackenbach, 1994; Vagero and Lundberg, 1989; and Fox et al., 1985.

Literatures concerning the economic returns to education are extensive and it is not the purpose of this paper to explore them. The issue of why these returns should be beneficial to health has received less attention. Two possible explanations are discussed here. One is that occupations requiring higher qualifications allow more occupational self-direction, which is related to self-efficacy and well-being and protects against depression (Kohn and Schooler, 1983; Kohn et al., 1990). English findings from a 20(+)-year follow-up to the Whitehall studies (Marmot et al., 1991) found that civil service employment grade was positively associated with greater self-efficacy and self-direction at work, more variety and challenge at work and greater job satisfaction. Those in higher grades also tended to report lower levels of hostility, fewer difficult life events, healthier lifestyles, and lower rates of morbidity. One explanation for these associations is that employment in higher grades is more fulfilling than employment in lower grades, and that this sense of fulfilment leads to lower levels of experienced stress and consequently lower rates of morbidity.

In contrast to these findings, analysis of the British Household Panel Survey (BHPS 1991 to 1997) suggests that the professional-managerial jobs that are associated with high levels of job satisfaction are also associated with high levels of stress (Rose, 2000). All other things being equal, one would expect this to lead to higher rates of morbidity (see p. 27).

A second possible mechanism through which economic returns to education are beneficial to health is that they provide protection against financial insecurity. Wilkinson (1996) suggests that for those with lower levels of qual-ifications, the detrimental effects of unemployment, low income and low occupational status upon health are psychosocially mediated through the stressors of job and financial insecurity. He cites evidence from numerous studies that the effects of economic deprivation upon health can be largely explained in terms of these psychosocial factors (Iverson and Klausen, 1981; Ferrie *et al.*, 1995; Cobb and Kasl, 1977; Mattiasson *et al.*, 1990; Ullah, 1990; Whelan, 1991).[1]

HEALTH-RELATED BEHAVIOURS

There is an extensive body of literature concerning health-related behaviours, their effects upon health, and the factors that predict them. This probably reflects an interest in the promotion of healthy behaviours.

Physical health-related behaviours of interest here include exercise, diet, dental hygiene, smoking, consumption of alcohol, consumption of other drugs, driving whilst intoxicated, use of seat belts, use of condoms, and adherence to medical advice. These behaviours appear to be positively correlated with one another (e.g. Costakis *et al.*, 1999; Feigelman *et al.*, 1998; Kyngas and Lahdenpera, 1999; Slater *et al.*, 1999; Thompson *et al.*, 1999).

There is abundant evidence that healthy behaviours impact upon physical and mental health. Some health-related behaviours, such as not wearing a seat belt, constitute a constant risk to health whilst others, such as smoking and excessive alcohol consumption, carry a cumulative risk. This latter group of behaviours rarely have immediate effects upon an individual's health, but additional years of smoking or heavy drinking are associated with higher risks to physical health later in life. The cumulative effects of health-related behaviours upon physical health may be one explanation for findings that the correlation between education and physical health is greater in magnitude amongst middle-aged and older populations than amongst younger people (Veenstra, 2000; Bynner and Egerton, 2001). An implication is that the observable effects of education upon young people are psychological and behavioural rather than physiological. In addition, correlations exist between health-related behaviours such as smoking, past substance abuse, and alcohol consumption and mental health (Kendler *et al.*, 1999).

It appears that years of education and level of qualification are positively associated with healthy behaviours. For example, studies report that individuals with more years of education and/or higher qualifications tend to exercise more, eat more nutritious and healthy diets, smoke less, give up smoking more, use condoms more, use seat belts more, and tend to comply better with medical instructions. The evidence also suggests that people with low levels of education are more likely to drink excessively and with intensity, or else to abstain from the consumption of alcohol. Details of the relevant studies are summarised in Table 4.

An additional outcome of education, which could be described as a health-related behaviour is cognitive activity in later years. This could provide an explanation for the observed correlation between years of formal education and lower rates of cognitive decline and Alzheimer's Disease amongst older people (Hall *et al.*, 1998; Breitner *et al.*, 1999). Certainly, there is evidence for an association between years of education and cognitive functioning in later life (Stevens *et al.* 1999; Viramo *et al.*, 1999; Deary *et al.*, 1998; Collie *et al.*, 1999; Weilgos and Cunningham 1999). This may be because those individuals who continue with post-compulsory education do so because they have a capacity and inclination to use their cognitive faculties, characteristics that are further developed through continued studying. Throughout the life course, these individuals will tend to obtain employment and seek out activities – such as leisure classes – that demand the use of their cognitive faculties. If this tendency continues into old age it is likely that the cognitive exercise may provide protection against cognitive decline, and ultimately against Alzheimer's Disease, just as regular physical activity affords protection against many physical conditions.

Like the correlation between learning and health, the correlation between learning and health-related behaviours may result from a variety of causes. Learning may promote healthy behaviours, but in addition, background variables like parental attitudes and lifestyles may incline individuals both to adopt healthy behaviours and to pursue their education, and healthy behaviours may play a role in the achievement of educational success and/ or the choice of educational path. Studies of the health-related behaviours of children and adolescents (ranging from smoking of cigarettes and marijuana, to use of other illegal drugs, heavy alcohol consumption, high-risk driving, and problem behaviours) make it clear that for these age groups at least, the relationships between learning and lifestyle are complex (e.g. Resnicow *et al.*, 1999; Koivusilta *et al.*, 1999; Provaznikova *et al.*, 1997; Karvonen *et al.*, 1999). Within this complex pattern of causation it is reasonable to suppose that the correlations between education and the adoption of healthy behaviours can be explained, in part at least, by the impact of learning upon health-related attitudes and behaviours. Indeed, there is evidence to support a number of mechanisms through which education affects health-related attitudes and behaviours. These mechanisms are outlined below.

Mediating factors between learning and health behaviours

Awareness

It appears that education increases awareness of information relevant to the adoption of a healthy lifestyle (e.g. Teisl *et al.*, 1999; Mirowsky and Ross, 1998). However, this awareness probably explains only a small part of the relationship between education and health-related behaviours. Using data from the Health Promotion/Disease Prevention Supplement to the 1985 National Health Interview Survey, Kenkel (1991) demonstrates that health knowledge about alcohol use, smoking and exercise only accounts for 5–20 per cent of the observed correlation between education and these behaviours (cited in Grossman and Kaestner, 1997). Perhaps this finding is not surprising. Marketing and advertising exploit the fact that our decisions are based upon hopes, dreams and fantasies, as well as the rational analysis of relevant information.

Future orientation

It has been suggested above (p. 11) that future-oriented thinking (that is, thinking within a long timescale, often referred to as time preference) may be a factor inclining individuals to invest in both education and a healthy lifestyle. This is a selection bias effect upon health. In addition, future orientation can be seen as a *mediating factor* between education and health-related behaviours – a social causation effect. Grossman and Kaestner (1997) quote Becker and Mulligan (1994), who argue that through the study of history, and through thinking about adulthood and imagined scenarios, pupils may learn to think in a future-oriented manner.

Evidence for associations between future orientation, education, and health outcomes come from two studies. Neither provides evidence to distinguish between the selection bias and social causation effects of future orientation upon health.

Based upon analyses of data from the USA, Kendler *et al.* (1999) report that nicotine dependence (but not smoking initiation) is related to a number of personality characteristics relating to future orientation: namely, mastery, self-esteem, locus of control, and dispositional optimism. Leigh and Dhir (1997) find an association between years of schooling and exercise amongst men living in the USA aged 65 and over, even after controlling for parental levels of education, family wealth during childhood, and area of residence during childhood. This association is partly but not entirely mediated by personality characteristics similar to those measured in Kendler's study – patience, self-efficacy, and risk preference.

Social effects

Recent health promotion initiatives the world over have placed increasing emphasis upon the importance of social norms and social attitudes in determining health-related behaviours. Examples include the National Healthy Schools Standard described above (p. 2) and peer programmes in developing countries, which draw upon Freire's notion of community empowerment through the development of critical awareness or consciousness. Evaluations of these programmes suggest that peer education is effective in changing health-related behaviours, although structural inequalities impose limitations (e.g., Campbell and Mzaidume, 2001; Campbell and Mzaidume, 2002).

The effectiveness of these programmes does not imply that mainstream education necessarily leads to the adoption of positive health-related behaviours, because we do not know which social values and social attitudes are promoted. Indeed, schools and colleges may be the environments where young adults first obtain and start using illegal drugs. Nevertheless, schools have tremendous potential to shape social values that can be health enhancing. This potential is recognised and built upon by the National Healthy Schools Standard.

In addition there is plenty of evidence that social support and connectedness are outcomes of learning (see Table 6 and p. 34 below), and also that social support per se reinforces healthy behaviours. Putnam reviews the evidence and suggests that socially isolated people are more likely to smoke, drink, overeat, and engage in other health-damaging behaviours (2000: 327).

Self-efficacy

As mentioned above, the Ottawa Charter for Health Promotion recognised that power and control were central issues in health promotion (Kickbusch, 1990). Thereafter, health promotion came to be widely understood as a process through which people are enabled to take control of their lifestyles and thereby improve their health (Whitty *et al.*, 1998).

Pearlin *et al.* (1981) define self-efficacy as, 'The extent to which people see themselves as being in control of the forces that importantly affect their lives'. This roughly equates with what Bandura calls *perceived* self-efficacy, which he suggests is concerned with judgements of personal capability (1997: 11). Perceived self-efficacy is a dynamic quality, which will vary throughout life.

Ross and Mirowsky describe how self-efficacy has a major impact upon health-related behaviours:

> The sense of personal control improves health partially through health-enhancing behaviours. Compared with people who feel powerless to control their lives, people with a sense of personal control know more about health, are more likely to initiate preventive behaviours like quitting smoking, exercising, or moderating alcohol consumption, and, in consequence, have better self-rated health, fewer illnesses, and lower rates of mortality (Seeman and Lewis 1995; Seeman and Seeman 1983; Seeman, Seeman, and Budros 1988). In contrast, lack of personal control makes efforts seem useless; if outcomes are beyond one's control, why exercise, quit smoking, or avoid overweight?
>
> (Ross and Mirowsky, 1999:446).

Numerous evaluations of health education programmes suggest that their effectiveness lies in changing health behaviours through empowering participants and building up their self-efficacy (e.g., Cable *et al.*, 1999; Barlow and Williams, 1999; Dusseldorp *et al.*, 1999).

Additional evidence suggests that higher levels of self-efficacy are associated with healthy behaviours – with respect to eating habits (Callaghan, 1998), freedom from nicotine dependence (Kendler *et al.*, 1999), adherence to treatments for kidney disease (Rudman *et al.*, 1999), and the monitoring of sugar intake and insulin levels to control diabetes (Rudman *et al.*, 1999).

If education generates self-efficacy, then this will act as a mediator between education and health-related behaviours. Mirowsky and Ross (1998) fit a covariate model to US data relating to over 2,500 adults, and find that 45 per cent of the association between education and health-related behaviours was mediated by a sense of personal control.

Self-efficacy appears to be an outcome of learning and education. Qualitative research exploring the immediate and delayed effects of education, and quantitative studies examining the relationships between education (measured by years of education and highest qualification) and hypothesised outcomes indicate that education generates self-efficacy across different types of learning provision (higher education, adult education, and learning through voluntary work), in different countries (USA, Britain), for different groups of learners (mature women, elders, people with mental health difficulties, and pregnant mothers), and for adults living in urban and rural areas at different stages in their lives. Details of the relevant studies are given in Table 5.

It is not difficult to think of reasons why education might generate self-efficacy. Within a context that is generally more flexible and supportive than the working environment, organised learning offers structure, purpose and a socially acceptable identity. These make a tremendous difference in terms of self-efficacy – and also self-esteem – for some groups, and are re-enforcing for all. Organised learning also sets challenges to each individual on the basis that the challenges will both stretch their capabilities and be met.

RESILIENCE AND DEALING WITH STRESS

Resilience refers to the dimension of individual difference that spans the ways we deal with adversity and stressful conditions and how they affect us (e.g., Garmezy, 1971; Anthony; 1974; Rutter, 1990).[2] The development of resilience in childhood has been examined fairly extensively. Howard *et al.*

(1999) have reviewed this literature and conclude that the internal assets that consistently describe the resilient child are autonomy, problem-solving skills, a sense of purpose and future, and social competence. They are developed in learning contexts that are integrated, co-operative, challenging, inclusive, heterogeneous, and that encourage participation and active learning (Benard, 1995; Frieberg *et al.*, 1995; Wang, 1997). A study of further education (FE) practitioners' views on wider benefits experienced by their students as a consequence of learning reports that some practitioners believe that increasing administrative burdens and overfull and inflexible curricula limit the extent to which they can sustain such a learning context (Preston and Hammond, 2002). Although such beliefs raise important issues, this aspect of the study used a non-representative sample of practitioners. In other words, we do not know how representative such views are amongst FE practitioners. Furthermore, they are perceptions only and may not be valid assessments.

The argument presented in this section is that although education can generate challenges, expectations, and lifestyles that are potentially stress-inducing, it can also broaden opportunities, provide security, and result in wider social support systems, and these can lead to ways of life that are less stress-inducing. In addition, education fosters qualities that contribute to resilience, which enables individuals to deal with stressful conditions and adversity without experiencing long-lasting stress. This is protective of both mental and physical health.

Intrinsic to the process of education is challenge. The nature and extent of challenges depends upon the learning experience, for example, methods of assessment and the competitiveness of the learning environment. These factors will determine the extent to which the challenges are stress-inducing.

Education also raises aspirations and expectations on the parts of students and their families and friends. Consequently, the degree of cognitive dissonance (i.e., the contrast between expectations and reality) that they are required to cope with if they fail to meet them is all the greater. In contrast with findings amongst the general population that more highly educated individuals experience lower rates of depression and better physical health, it appears that amongst the unemployed, those with higher qualifications are more likely to experience distress and develop depressive conditions and other physical health problems than those who are unemployed and have lower qualifications (Clark and Oswald, 1994; Turner, 1995).

Another way in which education can generate stress is through inclining those with high levels of qualifications towards employment and lifestyle options that may be fulfilling and are viewed as successful but that are nevertheless highly stress-inducing. As mentioned above (p. 20), Rose (2000) presents evidence based on data from the BHPS that higher stress occupations are mostly white-collar and from the professional-managerial employee strata, whilst low-stress occupations include craft skill groups, such as electricians, carpenters and plumbers, and other blue-collar workers.[3] These findings may reflect the way in which white-collar occupations have changed in the two decades since the Whitehall studies.

These hypothesised effects of education may account for the lack of consistent evidence for a correlation between education and rates of anxiety disorders reported above (p. 000). They might also contribute to explanations for the non-linearity of associations between qualification levels and depression found by Feinstein (2001) (see p. 13).

On the other hand, education broadens employment opportunities and provides security in ways that protect individuals from stressful conditions. This has been discussed on pp. 18–20. Moreover, the processes of education and learning develop many of the 'internal assets' that contribute towards resilience. These include self-efficacy, future orientation, inter-personal trust, anti-discriminatory attitudes, and social participation, discussed in the previous and following sections. Self-esteem, which is concerned with judgements of self-worth, may also play a part. Problem-solving also appears to be an outcome of both learning and education, since, as Mirowsky and Ross suggest, education 'instils the habit of meeting problems with attention, thought, action, and perseverance. [...] Education increases effort, which like ability is a fundamental component of problem solving (Wheaton, 1980)' (1998: 417).

If organised adult learning generates outcomes that build up an individual's resilience, enabling that individual to deal more effectively with adversity and stressful conditions, then this will not only relieve their distress. It will also contribute to better health. The relationship is perhaps most obvious in relation to depression since rates of depression are correlated with levels of self-esteem and self-efficacy (e.g., Battle,1978; Burnett and Mui, 1994; Turner and Turner, 1999).[4]

Numerous studies of students in community-based education who have a history of mental health difficulties report that participation has positive effects upon mental health (e.g. Wertheimer, 1997). Indeed, some GP practices now prescribe education as treatment for their patients (Wheeler *et al.*, 1999; James, 2001). Antikainen (1998) reports that some individuals find education and learning particularly empowering at times of transition, which are times of high stress relative to periods of stability.

In relation to the stresses induced by the process of education itself that were mentioned earlier, Bandura suggests that an individual's level of self-efficacy determines how they respond to pressures of academic demands. He argues that individuals with higher self-efficacy (a component of resilience) are less likely to become anxious and emotionally distressed in response to academic demands than individuals with lower levels of self-efficacy, regardless of their previous academic performances (1997: 235–7). This means that if education builds up an individuals' self-efficacy, this may help them to deal with the challenges that their education simultaneously presents. On the other hand, if learning takes place in a competitive environment that fosters neither personal development nor social cohesion, then it is easy to imagine that it could undermine self-efficacy and generate unhappiness and anxiety, leading to negative health outcomes.

To the extent that education builds resilience, this ability to deal effectively with adversity and stressful conditions will affect physical as well as mental health. Reliance upon nicotine, alcohol and other addictive substances as well as certain patterns of eating are sometimes responses to adversity and stressful conditions (e.g., Allison *et al.*, 1999). Individuals who through their education and learning feel independent and self-confident, who are used to solving problems, and who possess a sense of purpose and future may be inclined to respond in other ways which are less damaging to their health and possibly more effective in reducing levels of experienced stress in the longer term.

By definition, greater resilience results in lower levels of experienced chronic stress in response to a given stressor or life event. It is now well-established that whereas short-term stress responses may be essential for survival, long-lasting stress exacts a cost that can both promote the onset of illness and its progression (e.g. McEwan, 2000; Kubzansky *et al.*, 1999; Kiecolt-Glaser and Glaser, 1986. See also Wilkinson (1996: 179–81 for descriptions of a number of studies demonstrating that stress erodes physical health).[5]

In addition, levels of experienced stress and self-efficacy may affect the perception of certain symptoms such as pain. Several studies show that individuals with the same degree of tissue damage report different levels of pain (e.g. Beecher, 1956, cited in Ogden, 1997: 222–3). Turk *et al.* (1983, cited in Ogden 1997: 227) suggest that an individual's perception of pain is partially determined by their belief that they have control over the pain that they experience, as well as by levels of anxiety and neurosis (which are associated with experienced stress).

RELATIONSHIPS WITH MEDICAL PROFESSIONALS AND ACCESS TO MEDICAL SERVICES

Availability of and access to medical care tends to be lower amongst populations that are more deprived. These same populations are characterised by relatively high levels of poor health (e.g., Hart, 1971; Payne and Saul, 1997). For example, studies in Scotland suggest that patients who are socio-economically deprived, and who are thought to be particularly likely to develop coronary heart disease are less likely to be investigated and treated than their more socio-economically advantaged counterparts (Pell *et al.*, 2000; MacLeod *et al.*, 1999).[6] This ironic paradox that those most in need of medical support are least likely to receive it has been termed the 'inverse care law' (Hart, 1971).

Since those with more education tend to attain or maintain a relatively high socio-economic status, they will also tend to have better access to health care services. This may result partly from the effects of education upon understanding and evaluating the plethora of health and health service messages in the mass media, and partly from the ability to communicate effectively with health care professionals and elicit their help.

Where access to treatment or an acceptable diagnosis is denied, people who have more education are over-represented in pressure groups. These groups both reinforce individuals' attempts to obtain their medical rights and help to ensure that high quality services are made available to all. For example, a leading researcher and practitioner in CFS/ME states that 'too many studies to list show that the typical patient [with CFS/ME] joining a self-help organisation, comes from the upper social classes' (Wessely *et al.*, 1998: 147).

The effects of education and socio-economic status upon access to medical services is illustrated particularly sharply in relation to CFS/ME because it is a poorly understood condition. Studies of the prevalence rates of CFS/ME using samples taken from hospital clinics indicate a steep class gradient, the condition being apparently much more common amongst individuals of higher socio-economic status (Wessely *et al.*, 1998). However, community-based studies investigating the epidemiology of CFS/ME present a different picture, the class gradient being entirely absent (Buchwald *et al.*, 1995; Shefer *et al.*, 1997; Lawrie and Pelosi, 1995; Euba *et al.*, 1996). Wessely *et al.* (1998) suggest that this discrepancy in epidemiological findings between hospital-based and community-based studies reflects selection biases in how symptoms are attributed (e.g. to CFS/ME as opposed to depression or malingering), in diagnosis (e.g., of CFS/ME as opposed to depression or no diagnosis), and in referral for appropriate medical treatment. It is likely that the same could be true for other poorly understood conditions. For example, Heinrich *et al.* (1998) report higher rates of atopic disorders (which, like CFS/ME are poorly understood) amongst children whose parents have higher levels of education.

A patient's education may determine not only access to medical treatment but also its effectiveness. This is because patients with more education appear to be better informed and advised about the nature and management of their illnesses, and also tend to comply more with medical advice. For example, Rudman *et al.* (1999) surveyed almost 400 renal transplant patients in the USA and report that those with more years of education were more likely to comply with their post-trauma medical regimens. The association was small in magnitude, but statistically significant nevertheless. Peyrot *et al.* (1999) report similar findings in relation to glycemic control amongst just under 200 adult patients in Michigan (USA). Having a college education as opposed to not having one was associated with better chronic glycemic control for Type 1 diabetes. In addition, a survey of health service directors in the USA shows that they perceive typical recipients of screening programmes for cholesterol, breast cancer and cervical cancer to be adults with at least a high school education. A study outside the USA, of women living in Haifa (Israel) found that women who had participated in education for more years were more likely to initiate screening for breast cancer than women with fewer years of education, even after controlling for socio-economic status, age, and ethnicity (Hagoel *et al.*, 1999).

EDUCATION AND HEALTHY SOCIETIES

The relationship between an individual's socio-economic status and their health cannot be fully understood without reference to the society that they live in. In his seminal book , *Unhealthy Societies: The afflictions of inequality* (1996), Wilkinson concludes:

> In the developed world, it is not the richest countries which have the best health, but the most egalitarian. Having been demonstrated by a number of different people using different data sets and different control variables, this relationship is now firmly established.
>
> (Wilkinson, 1996: 3)

In other words, there is considerable evidence that above a basic threshold of national/regional financial security (referring mostly to developed as opposed to developing countries), health outcomes at national and regional levels are best predicted by relative as opposed to absolute levels of poverty. Nations, states, and communities characterised by high levels of financial inequality are characterised also by poorer general health outcomes and vice versa.

It has been suggested that nations/regions characterised by high levels of material inequality (in terms of income and security) are characterised also by inequality in educational opportunities as well as access to health and other welfare services (e.g. Wilkinson, 1996; Birdsall *et al.*, 1995). The causalities underlying connections between financial inequalities, educational opportunities and standards, and health are almost certainly complex. Wilkinson (1996) emphasises the effects of growing income disparity upon both health and educational standards. On the other hand, both Layard (1999) and Birdsall *et al.* (1995) suggest that income inequalities can be reduced through the provision of equal education to all. If this is correct, and equalising the provision of education decreases income inequalities, then there will be a positive knock-on effect upon health at national levels.

Layard compares the provision of equal education and cash redistribution as two hypothetical ways of reducing income disparity across a nation. He concludes that if income distribution is measured using measures of incomes over whole lifetimes as opposed to over a single year, then the equalising power of education is greater than that of cash redistribution. His argument assumes that family background and other characteristics have no effect upon returns from (equalised) schooling and that education costs nothing to the individual either directly through fees or indirectly through taxation. Birdsall *et al.* (1995) use statistics from the World Bank (1993) to suggest that reducing educational inequalities through investment in primary and secondary education in East Asian countries has resulted in a narrowing of income distributions and, incidentally, greater economic growth. The effect of equally accessible education upon income disparity is a mechanism through which the provision of a genuinely universal education could make people healthier at a national level.

Attempts to identify the means through which economic inequalities affect health at national levels have used the related concepts of social cohesion and social capital. The argument is based upon evidence for a close association between reduced income disparities and greater social cohesion and social capital – and vice versa. Wilkinson suggests that it is futile to attempt to separate out the directions of causality which account for this association. Rather, the two-way interactions between social and economic processes 'take place continuously throughout society with the occasional shifts one way or the other in the combined centre of gravity' (1996: 135).

Wilkinson's description of social cohesion emphasises the relevance of collective morality and social purpose to healthy societies. There is still no agreed definition of social capital, but one of the best known and most representative definitions can be found in the highly influential work of Putnam (1993):

> Social capital ... refers to features of social organisation, such as trust, norms, and networks, that can improve the efficiency of society by facilitating co-ordinated actions'
>
> (Putnam, 1993:167)

The most common measures of social capital look at participation in various forms of civic engagement, such as voter turnout and membership of voluntary organisations, and at levels of expressed trust in other people. The validity of these measures, and indeed of the concept of social capital is suggested by the high degree of correlation in country rankings on each of these variables, whilst showing wide inter-country variations on the aggregate social capital measures (Putnam, 2000).

There is a substantial literature demonstrating and investigating the positive effects of social capital, social cohesion, social connectedness, and social support upon physical and mental health. Longitudinal studies have been used to show that social isolation precedes illness, and that the effects of previous social isolation upon the incidence of illness persist after factors that may affect both social isolation and health are controlled for. In a chapter reviewing these effects, Putnam concludes that,

> Social connectedness is one of the most powerful determinants of our well-being. The more integrated we are with our community, the less likely we are to experience colds, heart attacks, strokes, cancer, depression, and premature death of all sorts.
>
> (Putnam, 2000: 326)

In addition, Gillies and Spray (1997) cite a number of health promotion projects based in disadvantaged communities in the UK. They suggest that building local networks and institutions, and promoting volunteer activities and peer programmes with the direct involvement of local people, can have relatively speedy health benefits.

We have here an argument based upon empirical evidence – albeit an argument that involves a chain of causalities – for a mechanism through which the provision of education that is genuinely equal has a positive effect upon a nation's health. The chain of causalities begins with the effects of reduced educational inequalities upon narrowing income distributions, and continues with the positive effects of narrowed income distributions upon social cohesion and social capital, and the effects of social cohesion and social capital upon health. It is also likely that the equalising participation in education has direct effects upon social cohesion. This argument is illustrated in Figure 3.

What is meant by equalising participation in education, and how this can best be achieved in Britain, are important questions that are investigated elsewhere (McGivney, 2001; Haggart, 2001; Beinart and Smith (1997). Birdsall *et al.* (1995) examine the effects of different education policies across different countries and suggest that an effective means of equalising educational experiences (and consequently, income distributions) in East Asian countries has been heavy investment in primary and secondary education. There are a number of policies in Britain and other countries that target educational provision towards adults with few or no qualifications.

The preceding discussion has been concerned with the effects of equalising education across nations upon social cohesion. In addition, education can be used to build social cohesion at a local level and consequently improve the health of individuals and communities. This vision is expanded upon in the paper by Whitty and colleagues (1998), and motivates educational interventions aimed at reducing health inequalities, for example, those organised through Health Action Zones and Health Improvement Projects (see pp. 1–2).

In relation to more mainstream education, there is strong evidence that social capital correlates with education at the level of the individual. In a recent paper concerning the formation of social capital, Glaeser (2000) reviews evidence from the General Social Survey in the USA, and the international World Values Survey, and concludes, 'There is no more robust correlate of social capital variables than years of schooling' (5).

One explanation for this correlation is that many of the immediate outcomes of education and learning are defining qualities of social capital and social cohesion. These outcomes include inter-personal trust, anti-discriminatory attitudes, supportive relationships, voluntary activity, connectedness and a sense of community. The evidence is summarised in Table 6. It has been suggested earlier that these same outcomes are likely to reinforce healthy behaviours, reduce levels of chronic stress, and ensure access to medical services (see pp. 14, 27 and 29). Interestingly, Putnam suggests identical explanations for why social capital matters for health, adding that social networks may furnish tangible assistance, such as money, convalescent care, and transportation. This suggests that social capital describes a combination of the outcomes of learning which, operating at an aggregate level, have healthy effects upon whole communities.

Chapter 4

Conclusions

There is a substantial body of evidence suggesting that positive correlations exist between education and physical and mental health. There are multiple explanations for these observed correlations. It appears that some factors such as family background and future orientation affect both educational level achieved and health outcomes. In addition, there is evidence that health status affects educational outcomes. The third explanation is that education has effects upon health.

The purpose of this paper has been to investigate the third of these explanations by examining the evidence for a variety of mechanisms through which learning and education affect health. A theme which emerges from discussion of the mechanisms is that the immediate outcomes of education play a fundamental role in generating the behaviours, skills and personal attributes that have early but lasting effects upon mental health and cumulative effects upon physical health. This is illustrated in the model of the mechanisms through which learning affects health in Figure 1.

Immediate outcomes of education are often dynamic and inter-related, and include increased levels of self-esteem, self-efficacy, problem-solving skills, aspirations, future orientation, inter-personal trust, social competence, anti-discriminatory attitudes, and a feeling of belonging. Such outcomes reflect the deeply empowering and socialising potential of education. They generate personal resilience, healthy lifestyles, successful access to medical services, and economic success – all of which have beneficial effects upon psychological and physiological health. In addition, the social outcomes of education appear to raise indicators of social capital, and it has been shown that social capital has positive effects upon the health of whole communities.

It appears that social capital can be developed not only through raising levels of education amongst individuals but also through reducing educational inequalities across individuals. It is suggested that reducing inequalities in educational experiences may reduce disparities in income and have positive effects not only upon social cohesion but also upon health. Of course, increases in social capital have other positive effects, such as reduced crime rates and active ageing (e.g., Putnam, 2000).

A paradox is the lack of consistent evidence for correlations between education and happiness and between education and anxiety disorders. One explanation is that learning alone cannot guarantee these outcomes, but learning in combination with other things such as social capital and appropriate opportunities for progression and employment probably does.

If education plays such an important role in promoting mental and physical health at individual and community levels, then this is a strong and clear message that policies about the provision and promotion of lifelong learning have tremendous relevance to building up the health of the nation. One implication concerns the importance of genuinely universal provision of education and raises questions about how this can be achieved. Another is the need for further analysis of the effects of different forms of learning in different contexts to inform policies about the aspects of education that result in improvements in health.

Table 1 Summary of the evidence for positive correlations between education and physical health in different countries

Geographical locations where correlations were found	References to studies
Worldwide	McMahon, 1999
Developing countries	World Bank, 1993 Rodrigues-Garcia and Goldman, 1994
Throughout the USA	Desai, 1987 Gilleskie and Harrison, 1998 Pappas *et al.*, 1993 Ross and Mirowsky, 1999
Canada	Veenstra, 2000
Quebec	Noreau *et al.*, 1999
Australia	National Health Strategy, 1992 Benzeval *et al.*, 1995 Mitchell *et al.*, 1997
Italy	Piperno and Di Orio, 1990 Benzeval *et al.*, 1995 Varenna *et al.*, 1999
Britain	Montgomery and Schoon, 1997
The Netherlands	Mackenbach, 1993 Benzeval *et al.*, 1995
Sweden	Wamala *et al.*, 1999
Finland	Valkonen, 1993 Benzeval *et al.*, 1995 Sihvonen *et al.*, 1998
Norway	Sihvonen *et al.*, 1998

Table 2 Summary of the evidence for positive correlations between education and physical health amongst different groups of individuals and over a range of health outcomes

Groups of individuals amongst whom the correlation was found	Health outcomes that correlate with education	References to studies
American Indians in the USA	Depression and subjective well-being following spinal injuries	Krause *et al.*, 1999
African-Americans over 65	Alzheimer's Disease	Hall *et al.*, 1998
High-income group white males in the USA	Mortality rates and self-rated health	Grossman, 1975
Low-income working males in the USA	Self-rated health and number of days off work due to sickness	Desai, 1987
Older men aged 60 to 67 across income, marital status, and input health	Self-rated health	Taubman and Rosen, 1982
Men and women aged 50 to 94 in Australia	Self-rated general, physical and mental health	Mitchell *et al.*, 1997
Middle and older age groups in Canada. No correlation found amongst younger people	Self-rated health status	Veenstra, 2000
Men aged 70+ in the USA. The relationship was not statistically significant amongst women of this age group	Risk of hospitalisation for acute myocardial infarction	Wolinsky *et al.*, 1999
Elderly community residents in Utah, USA.	Alzheimer's Disease	Breitner *et al.*, 1999
Postmenopausal women living in Italy	Prevalence of osteoporosis	Varenna *et al.*, 1999
Adult women up to 65 living in Sweden	Coronary heart disease	Wamala *et al.*, 1999
70- to 79-year-olds functioning above average physically and cognitively in the USA	Decreased pulmonary function, increased body mass index	Kubzansky *et al.*, 1998
Adults living in the USA	Chronic fatigue	Clark *et al.*, 1995
Scotland	Chronic fatigue	Lawrie and Pelosi, 1995

Table 3 Summary of the evidence for a correlation between (more) education and (lower) rates of depressive conditions

Groups of individuals amongst whom the correlation was found	Health outcomes that correlate with education	References to studies
Cohort born in Britain in 1970	Rates of depression	Montgomery and Schoon, 1997
Frail elderly living alone in the USA	Rates of depression	Burnette and Mui, 1994
Puerto Ricans in New York City	Rates of depression	Potter *et al.*, 1995
Random sample of older people (mean age 74.2) with a hearing impairment in Southern Italy	Rates of depression	Cacciatore *et al.*, 1999
Random sample of Chinese people aged 65+ living in Singapore	Rates of depressive conditions co-morbid with other psychiatric disorders, predominantly anxiety	Heok *et al.*, 1996
Mothers in East Turkey	Postpartum psychosis	Kirpinar *et al.*, 1999[7]
Mothers in Peru	Postpartum depression	Vega Dienstmaier *et al.*, 1999
Australian former army conscripts of the Vietnam conflict era	Suicide	O'Toole and Cantor, 1995
Young adults living in rural and urban areas of Spain	Suicide attempts	Ferrero *et al.*, 1994[8]
Inuit aged 14–25 years residing in a community in Northern Quebec	Suicide attempts	Kirmayer *et al.*, 1996[9]
Community sample of older adolescents in the USA	Suicide attempts	Andrews and Lewinsohn, 1992
Nationally representative sample in the USA	Self-rated satisfaction with life	Putnam, 2000

Table 4 Summary of the evidence for positive correlations between education and health-related behaviours

Health-related behaviour that is positively correlated with level of education	Reference
Physical exercise	Frisk *et al.*, 1997 Wadsworth *et al.*, 1997 Ross and Mirowsky, 1999 Kubzansky *et al.*, 1999
Healthy diet / not overweight	Braddon *et al.*, 1988 Ippolito and Mathius, 1990 Wadsworth *et al.*, 1997 Schafer *et al.*, 1999
Smoke less	Kubzansky *et al.*, 1999 Sander, 1995a Wadsworth *et al.*, 1997 Kendler *et al.*, 1999 Jorm *et al.*, 1999
Give up smoking	Sander, 1995b
Alcohol consumption that is not excessive or intense, but may be frequent	Van Oers *et al.*, 1999 Berggren and Sutton, 1999
Not abstaining from alcohol	Van Oers *et al.*, 1999 Ross and Mirowsky, 1999
Use of condoms	Kasenda *et al.*, 1997
Use of seat belts	Leigh, 1990
Compliance with medical instructions	Hagoel *et al.*, 1999 Amonkar *et al.*, 1999 Kyngas and Lahdenpera, 1999 Peyrot *et al.*, 1999 Rudman *et al.*, 1999

Table 5 **Details of studies that demonstrate that self-efficacy and self-esteem are outcomes of learning**

Outcome of learning	Type of learning provision	Details of learners	Country	Approach used	Reference
A new sense of self-evaluation and individuality	Higher education	Mature women	England	Individual depth interviews	Cox and Pascall, 1994
Coherence	Access courses and higher education	Adults	England	Qualitative	West, 1995
Confidence, ability to cope with everyday life	All types	Adults	England and Wales	Survey plus Depth interviews	Dench and Regan, 1999
Increased confidence and self-esteem	Informal learning	Older adults	Britain	Qualitative	Carlton and Soulsby, 1999
Increased confidence, empowerment	Courses provided by colleges in the community	People experiencing mental health difficulties	England and Wales	Review of various studies	Wertheimer, 1997
Increased confidence, empowerment	Various	Long-term unemployed, people with long-term health and disability problems or mental health problems, isolated, elderly.	Gloucester, England	Evaluation of a project	McGivney, 199
Increased self-efficacy, mastery and happiness	Level of previous education	Older people who are physically and cognitively fit	USA	Quantitative using in-home interviews	Kubzansky *et al.*, 1999
Empowerment	All forms of planned learning	People living in rural and urban areas and at different stages in their lives	Finland	Qualitative biographical methods	Antikainen, 1998

cont'd

Table 5 **Details of studies that demonstrate that self-efficacy and self-esteem are outcomes of learning** *(cont'd)*

Outcome of learning	Type of learning provision	Details of learners	Country	Approach used	Reference
Increased self-esteem[10]	Mentees in a psychosocial support programme	Older adults	USA	Self-completion questionnaire	Koberg *et al.*, 1998
Increased self-esteem	Level of previous education	White and Hispanic pregnant women	USA	Quantitative: interviews and questionnaires	Rini *et al.*, 1999
Increased self-esteem	'New beginnings' courses	Adults	England	Interviews and questionnaires	Hull, 1998
Perceived happiness	Current education	Older adults	USA	Qualitative	Mookherjee, 1998

Table 6 **Summary of some of the literature that suggests that outcomes of learning include defining qualities of social capital**

Outcome of learning	Measurement used for learning	Category of learner	Methodological approach	Reference
Social capital	Various	Various	Review	Glaeser, 1999
Empathy building and a sense of community	Mainstream 'intermediate' level	US secondary school students	Analysis of minutes of meetings	Angell, 1998
	Various	People with mental health difficulties living in England and Wales	Review	Wertheimer, 1997
	Participation in a variety of educational provision	People with mental health difficulties living in Gloucester, England	Evaluation of a programme	McGivney, 1997
	Community-based physical education programme entitled 'Sport for Peace'	US high school students	Observation and interviews	Ennis *et al.*, 1999
Connectedness and a broader outlook	Attendance at a Summer University	Older learners in Britain	Qualitative	Jarvis and Walker, 1997
	Participation in a variety of educational provision	People with mental health difficulties living in Gloucester, England	Evaluation of a programme	McGivney, 1997
	Years of formal education and level of attainment	Various	Review	Emler and Frazer, 1999
Lower rates of ethnic prejudice using subtle measures	Years of formal education	Representative of Europeans	Analysis of data from Eurobarometer and qualitative	Wagner and Zick, 1995
Inter-personal trust	Higher Education	Nationally representative sample of British adults born in 1958	Secondary analysis	Bynner and Egerton, 2001
Lowered levels of hostility	Level of education	Community-dwelling men in Greater Boston area, US, aged 51+	Secondary analysis	Kubzansky *et al.*, 1999

cont'd

Table 6 Summary of some of the literature that suggests that outcomes of learning include defining qualities of social capital *(cont'd)*

Outcome of learning	Measurement used for learning	Category of learner	Methodological approach	Reference
Supportive relationships	Years of schooling, college degree, academic quality of the school	Nationally representative sample of US adults	Secondary analysis	Ross and Mirowsky, 1999
	Mentoring on a health education course	People aged 55+ living in the Netherlands	Quasi-experimental evaluation using questionnaire	Kocken and Voorham, 1998
	Higher Education	Nationally representative sample of British adults born in 1958.	Secondary analysis	Bynner and Egerton, 2001
Voluntary activity	Higher Education	Adults in Britain	Secondary analysis	Parry *et al.*, 1992
	Various	Various	Review	Emler and Frazer, 1999
Political engagement, activity, and identity.	Education of parents and educational success before age of 20	Young adults in Britain	Secondary analysis of longitudinal datasets	Bynner and Ashford, 1994
	Higher Education	Nationally representative sample of British adults born in 1958	Secondary analysis	Bynner and Egerton, 2001

Figure 1 **Model of the mechanisms through which learning affects health**

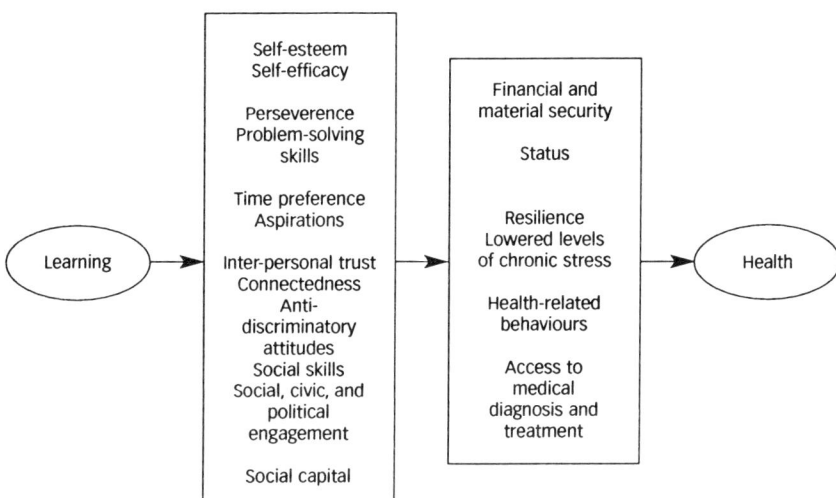

Figure 2 **Three explanations for the observed positive correlations between education and health**

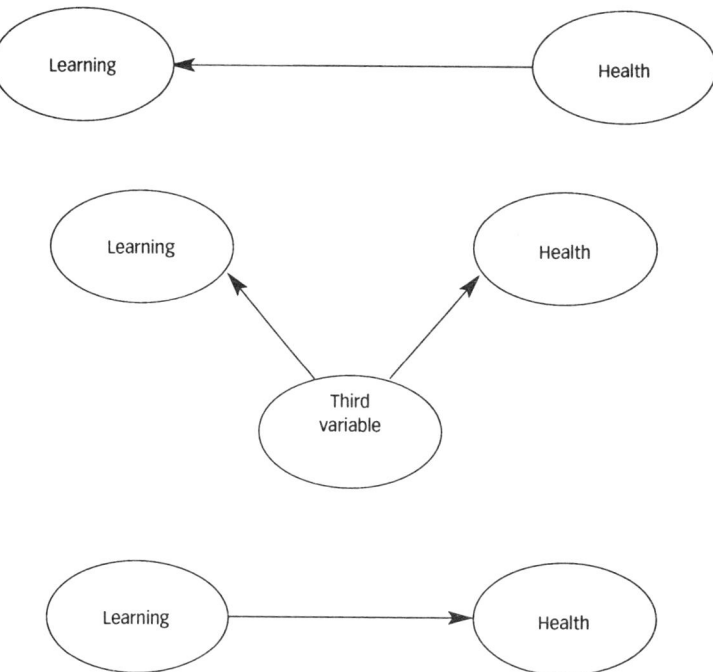

Figure 3 **Some relationships between educational disparities, income disparities and health**

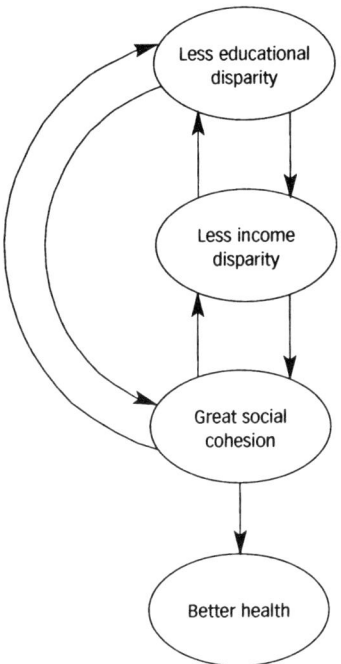

Notes

1 Wilkinson is careful to emphasise that his discussion of psychological pathways does not mean that the basic cause of the problem is psychological or can be dealt with by psychological interventions (184).

2 It may be helpful to distinguish between the terms 'stressful conditions', otherwise referred to a 'stressor', and 'experienced stress', referred to also as 'distress'. In a textbook of health psychology, Ogden defines stress in the following way: 'Contemporary definitions of stress regard the external environmental stress as a stressor (e.g. problems at work), the response to the stressor as stress or distress (e.g. the feeling of tension) and the concept of stress as something which involves biochemical, physiological, behavioural and psychological changes' (Ogden, 1997 : 201).

3 Levels of experienced stress are measured using self-report and this measure is validated against other more objective measures such as

blood pressure, digestion, rates of acute episodes of anxiety and depression, and migraine.

4 The directions of causality are not clear. Low self-esteem and self-efficacy may predispose individuals to develop depressive conditions, but they are also symptoms of depression.

5 Ogden (1997: 210) suggests that stress may be related to illness via the following physiological pathways:

- stress may cause an increase in acid secretion in the stomach, which may cause ulcers
- stress may result in increased cardiovascular response, and increased chances of injury or damage to arteries via plaque formation and fat deposits
- stress is hormonally mediated by the production of catecholamines, which can raise the chances of blood clot formation and consequently of heart attack
- high levels of catecholamines can also lead to kidney disease
- high levels of catecholamines and corticosteroids (another hormonal mediator of stress) affect the immune system making the individual more susceptible to infection
- high levels of corticosteroids can lead to arthritis.

6 But see Richards et al., 2000, who found no evidence for social differences in patient presentation or general practitioner diagnoses that might have explained differential uptakes of cardiovascular services.

7 The sample size for this study is 64 and no conclusions about statistic significance can be drawn. However, the majority of patients with postpartum psychosis had a low educational level.

8 The sample size was 100.

9 The sample size for this study was 99, which means that the statistical significance of findings may not be altogether reliable.

10 Self-esteem is measured using four bipolar descriptions: successful/not successful, important/not important, doing my best/not doing my best, happy/sad. The first three of these items could be interpreted as measuring self-efficacy rather than self-worth.

Bibliography

Acheson, D. (1998) 'Independent inquiry into inequalities in health'. London: The Stationery Office.

Allison, K.R., Adlaf, E.M., Ialomiteanu, A. and Rehm, J. (1999) 'Predictors of health risk behaviours among young adults: analysis of the national population health survey'. *Canadian Journal of Public Health*, 90 (2): 85–9.

Amonkar, M.E., Madhavan, S., Rosenbluth, S.A. and Simon, K.J. (1999) 'Barriers and facilitators to providing common preventive screening services in managed care settings'. *Journal of Community Health*, 24 (3): 229–47.

Andrews, J.A. and Lewinsohn, P.M. (1992) 'Suicidal attempts among older adolescents – prevalence and concurrence with psychiatric disorders'. *Journal of the American Academy of Child and Adolescent Psychiatry*, 31 (4): 655–62.

Angell, A.V. (1998) 'Practicing democracy at school: a qualitative analysis of an elementary class council'. *Theory and Research in Social Education*, 26 (2): 149–72.

Anthony, E.J. (1974) 'The syndrome of the psychologically invulnerable child'. In E.J. Anthony and C. Koupernik (eds) 'The child in his family: children at psychiatric risk'. *International Yearbook*, Vol. 3. New York: Wiley.

Antikainen, A. (1998) 'Between structure and subjectivity: life-histories and lifelong learning'. *International Review of Education*, 44 (2–3): 215–34.

Arnarson, E.O., Gudmundsdottir A. and Boyle, G.J. (1998) 'Six-month prevalence of phobic symptoms in Iceland: an epidemiological postal survey'. *Journal of Clinical Psychology*, 54 (2): 257–65.

Asplund, R. and Pereira, P. (1999) *Returns to Human Capital in Europe: A literature review*. Helsinki: ETLA, The Research Institute of the Finnish Economy/Taloustieto Oy.

Bandura, A. (1997) *Self-Efficacy: The exercise of control*. New York: W.H. Freeman.

Banks, M., Bates, I., Breakwell, G., Bynner, J., Emler, N., Jamieson, L. and Roberts, K. (1992) *Careers and Identities*. Milton Keynes: Open University Press.

Barlow, J.H. and Williams, B. (1999) 'I now feel that I'm not just a bit of left luggage': the experiences of older women with arthritis attending a personal independence course'. *Disability and Society*, 14 (1): 53–64.

Battle, J. (1978) 'Relationship between self-esteem and depression'. *Psychological Reports*, 42: 745:6.

Becker, G.S. (1993) *Human Capital: A theoretical and empirical analysis, with special reference to education* (3rd edn). Chicago: University of Chicago Press.

Becker, G.S. and Mulligan, C.B. (1994) 'On the endogenous determination of time preference'. *Discussion paper 94-2*, Chicago: Economics Research Center/National Opinion Research Center, Mimeo.

Beecher, H.K. (1956) 'Relationship of significance of wound to the pain experienced'. *Journal of the American Medical Association*, 161: 1609–13.

Beekman, A.T.F., Bremmer, M.A., Deeg, D.J.H., van Balkom, A.J.L.M., Smit, J.H., de Beurs, E., van Dyke, R. and van Tilburg, W. (1998) 'Anxiety disorder in later life: a report from the longitudinal aging study Amsterdam'. *International Journal of Geriatric Psychiatry*, 13 (10): 717–26.

Behrman, J.R. and Wolfe, B.L. (1989) 'Does schooling make a woman better nourished and healthier? Adult sibling random and fixed effects estimates for Nicaragua'. *Journal of Human Resources*, 24: 644–63.

Beinart, S. and Smith, P. (1998) 'National Adult Learning Survey 1997'. Research Report 49. London: DfEE.

Benard, B. (1995) 'Fostering resilience in children. ERIC/EECE Digest, EDO-PS-95-9.

Benham, L. and Benham, A. (1982) 'Employment, earnings, and psychiatric diagnosis'. In V.R. Fuchs (ed.), *Economic Aspects of Health*. NBER: University of Chicago Press: 202–20.

Benzeval, M., Judge, K. and Whitehead, M. (1995) 'Introduction'. In M. Benzeval, K. Judge and M. Whitehead (eds), *Tackling Inequalities in Health: An agenda for action*. London: King's Fund.

Berggren, F. and Sutton, M. (1999) 'Are frequency and intensity of participation decision-bearing aspects of consumption? An analysis of drinking behaviour'. *Applied Economics*, 31 (7): 865–74.

Bergman, A.J. and Walker, E. (1995) 'The relationship between cognitive functions and behavioural deviance in children at risk for psychopathology'. *Journal of Child Psychology and Psychiatry and Allied Disciplines*, 36 (2): 265–78.

Birdsall, N., Ross, D. and Sabot, R. (1995) 'Inequality and growth reconsidered – lessons from East Asia'. *World Bank Economic Review*, 9 (3): 477–508.

Black, D., Morris, J., Smith, C., Townsend, P., edited by Peter Townsend and Nick Davidson (1982) *Inequalities in Health – The Black Report*. Harmondsworth: Penguin.

Braddon, F.E.M., Wadsworth, M.E.J., Davies, J.M.C. and Cripps, H.A. (1988) 'Social and regional differences in food and alcohol consumption and their measurement in a National Birth Cohort'. *Journal of Epidemiology and Community Health*, 42: 341–49.

Breitner, J.C.S., Wyse, B.W., Anthony, J.C., Welsh Bohmer, K.A., Steffens, D.C., Norton, M.C., Tschanz, J.T., Plassman, B.L., Meyer, M.R., Skoog, I. and Khachaturian, A. (1999) 'APOE-epsilon 4 count predicts age when prevalence of AD increases, then declines – The Cache County Study'. *Neurology*, 53 (2): 321–31.

Buchwald, D., Umali, P., Umali, J., Kith, P., Pearlman, T. and Komaroff, A. (1995) 'Chronic fatigue and the chronic fatigue syndrome: prevalence in a Pacific Northwest Health Care System'. *Annals of Internal Medicine*, 123: 81–8.

Burnette, B. and Mui, A.C. (1994) 'Determinants of self-reported depressive symptoms by frail elderly persons living alone'. *Journal of Gerontological Social Work*, 22 (1–2): 3–19.

Bynner, J. and Ashford, S. (1994) 'Politics and participation: some antecedents of young people's political activity and disaffection'. *European Journal of Social Psychology*, 24: 223–26.

Bynner, J. and Egerton, M. (2001) 'The wider benefits of higher education'. Report 01/46. Bristol: HEFCE.

Bynner, J. and Roberts, K. (1991) *Youth and Work: Transition to employment in England and Germany*. London: Anglo German Foundation.

Cable, T.A., Meland, E., Soberg, T. and Slagsvold S. (1999) 'Lessons from the Oslo study diet and anti-smoking trial: a qualitative study of long-term behaviour change'. *Scandinavian Journal of Public Health*, 27 (3): 206–12.

Cacciatore, F., Napoli, C., Abete, P., Marciano, E., Triassi, M. and Rengo, F. (1999) 'Quality of life determinants and hearing function in an elderly population: Osservatorio Geriatrico Campano study group'. *Gerontology*, 45 (6): 323–8.

Callaghan, P. (1998) 'Social support and locus of control as correlates of UK nurses' health-related behaviours'. *Journal of Advanced Nursing*, 28 (5): 1127–33.

Campbell, C. and Mzaidume, Z. (2001) 'Grassroots participation, peer education, and HIV prevention by sex workers in South Africa'. *American Journal of Public Health*, 91 (12): 1978–86.

Campbell, C. and Mzaidume, Z. (2002) 'How can HIV be prevented in South Africa? A social perspective'. *British Medical Journal*, 324: 229–32.

Cannon, M., Jones, P., Gilvarry, C., Rifkin, L., McKenzie, K., Foerster, A. and Murray, R.M. (1997) 'Premorbid social functioning in schizophrenia and bipolar disorder: similarity and differences'. *American Journal of Psychiatry*, 154 (11): 1544–50.

Carlton, S. and Soulsby, J. (1999) *Learning to Grow Older and Bolder*. Leicester: NIACE.

Chaikind, S. and Corman, H. (1991) 'The impact of low birthweight on special education costs'. *Journal of Health Economics*, 10: 291–311.

Chevalier, A., Lanot, G., Walker, I. And Woolley, P. (1999) 'The Returns to Education in the UK'. In Asplund, R. and Pereira, P. (eds) *Returns to Human Capital in Europe: A literature review*. Helsinki: ETLA, The Research Institute of the Finnish Economy/Taloustieto Oy: 351–67.

Clark, M.R., Katon, W., Russo, J., Kith, P., Sintay, M. and Buchwald, D. (1995)

'Chronic fatigue – risk-factors for symptom persistence in a ½ year follow-up study'. *American Journal of Medicine*, 98 (2): 187–95.

Clark, A.E. and Oswald, A.J. (1994) 'Unhappiness and unemployment'. *Economic Journal*, 104: 648–9.

Cobb, S. and Kasl, S.C. (1977) 'Termination: the consequences of job loss'. Cincinnati: Department of Health, Education and Welfare/US National Institutes for Occupational Safety and Health, publication no. 77-224.

Collie A., ShafiqAntonacci R., Maruff, P., Tyler, P. and Currie, J. (1999) 'Norms and the effects of demographic variables on a neuropsychological battery for use in healthy ageing Australian populations.' *Australian and New Zealand Journal of Psychiatry*, 33 (4): 568–75.

Corman, H. and Grossman, M. (1985) 'Determinants of neonatal mortality rates in the United States.: a reduced form model'. *Journal of Health Economics*, 4: 213–36.

Costakis, C.E., Dunnagan, T. and Haynes, G. (1999) 'The relationship between stages of exercise adoption and other health behaviors'. *American Journal of Promotion*, 14 (1): 22–30.

Cox, R. and Pascall, G. (1994) 'Individualism, self-evaluation and self-fulfilment in the experience of mature women students'. *International Journal of Lifelong Education*, 13 (2): 159–73.

Deary, I.J., MacLennan, W.J. and Starr, J.M. (1998) 'Is age kinder to the initially more able? Differential ageing of a verbal ability in the healthy old people in Edinburgh study'. *Intelligence* , 26 (4): 357–75.

Dench, S. and Regan, J. (1999) 'Learning in later life: motivation and impact'. Report issued by the Institute for Employment Studies, Brighton.

Desai, S. (1987) 'The estimation of the health-production function for low-income working men.' *Medical Care*, 25: 604–15.

DfEE (1998) *The Learning Age: A renaissance for a new Britain*. Green Paper. London: The Stationery Office.

Dusseldorp, E., van Eldoren, T., Maes, S., Meulen, Kraaij (1999) 'A meta-analysis of psychoeducational programs for coronary heart disease patients'. *Health Psychology*, 18 (5): 506–19.

Edwards, L.N, and Grossman, M. (1979) 'The relationship between children's health and intellectual development'. In S.J. Mushkin and D.W. Dunlop (eds) *Health: What is it worth*. Elmsford: Pergamon Press.

Emler, N. and Frazer, E. (1999) 'Politics, the education effect'. *Oxford Review of Education*. 25 (1 and 2): 251–73.

Ennis, C.D., Solmon, M.A., Satina, B., Loftus, S.J., Mensch, J. and McCauley, M.T. (1999) 'Creating a sense of family in urban schools using the "Sport for Peace" curriculum'. *Research Quarterly for Exercise and Sport*, 70 (3): 273–85.

Esping-Anderson, G. (1993) *Changing Classes: Stratification and mobility in post-industrialist societies*. Sage: London.

Euba, R., Chalder, T., Deale, A. and Wessely, S. (1996) 'A comparison of the characteristics of chronic fatigue syndrome in primary and tertiary care'. *British Journal of Psychiatry*, 168 (121):6.

Farrell, P. and Fuchs, V.R. (1982) 'Schooling and health: the cigarette connection'. *Journal of Health Economics*, 1: 217–30.

Feigelman, W., Wallisch, L.S. and Lesieur, H.R. (1998) 'Problem gamblers, problem substance users, and dual-problem individuals: An epidemiological study'. *American Journal of Public Health*, 88 (3): 467–70.

Feinstein, L. (2001) 'Review of quantified evidence on the wider benefits of learning and related potential costs and savings: crime and health'. Unpublished report by the Centre for Research on the Wider Benefits of Learning to the DfES.

Ferrero, V., Marco, G., Benitez, H., Derivera, G. and Revuela, J.L. (1994) 'Risk-factors in suicide attempts'. *Folia Neuropsiquiatrica*, 29: 35–54.

Ferrie, J.E., Shipley, M.J., Marmot, M.G., Stansfield, S. and Davey Smith, G. (1995) 'Health effects of anticipation of job change and non-employment: longitudinal data from the Whitehall II study'. *British Medical Journal*, 311: 1264–9.

Fox, A.J., Moser, K.A., Jones, D.R. and Goldblatt, P.O. (1985) 'Socio-demographic differentials in mortality, 1971–81'. *Population Trends*, 40: 10–16.

Freiberg, H.J., Stein, T.A. and Huang, S.L. (1995) 'The effects of classroom management intervention on student achievement in inner city elementary schools'. *Educational Research and Evaluation*, 1 (1): 33–66.

Frisk, J., Brynhildsen, J., Ivarsson, T., Persson, P. and Hammar, M. (1997) 'Exercise and smoking habits among Swedish postmenopausal women'. *British Journal of Sports Medicine*, 31 (3): 217–23.

Fuchs, V.R. (1982) 'Time preference and health: an exploratory study'. In V.R. Fuchs (ed.), *Economic Aspects of Health*. Chicago: University of Chicago Press.

Garmezy, N. (1971) 'Vulnerability research and the issue of primary prevention'. *Journal of Orthopsychiatry*, 41:101–16.

Gilleskie, D.B. and Harrison, A. L. (1998) 'The effect of endogenous health inputs on the relationship between health and education'. *Economics of Education Review*, 17 (3): 279–96.

Gillies, P. and Spray, J. (1997) *Addressing Health Inequalities: The practical potential of social capital*. London: Health Education Authority.

Glaeser, E.L. (2000) 'The formation of social capital'. Paper delivered at OECD/Canada Statistics Conference on Human and Social Capital, Quebec.

Glewwe, P. (1997) *How does Schooling of Mothers Improve Child Health? Evidence from Morocco*. Living Standards Measurement Working Paper, 128. Washington, DC: World Bank.

Grossman, M. (1975) 'The correlation between health and schooling'. In N.E. Terleckyj (ed.), *Household Production and Consumption: Studies in income and wealth*. Conference on Research in Income and Wealth. New York: Columbia University Press for the National Bureau of Economic Research.

Grossman, M. and Joyce, T.M. (1990) 'Unobservables, pregnancy resolutions, and birth weight production functions in New York City'. *Journal of Political Economy*, 98: 983–1007.

Grossman, M. and Kaestner, R. (1997) 'Effects of education on health'. In J.R. Behrman and N. Stacey (eds), *The Social Benefits of Education*. Ann Arbor: University of Michigan Press.

Haggart, J. (2001). *Walking Ten Feet Tall: A toolkit for family learning practitioners*. London: DfES and NIACE.

Hagoel L., Ore, L., Neter, E., Shifroni, G. and Rennert G. (1999) 'The gradient in mammography screening behavior: a lifestyle marker'. *Social Science and Medicine*, 48 (9): 1281–90.

Hall, K., Gureje, O., Gao, S., Ogunniyi, A., Hui, S.L., Baiyewu, O., Unverzagt, F.W., Oluwole, S. and Hendrie, H.C. (1998) 'Risk factors and Alzheimer's disease: a comparative study of two communities'. *Australian and New Zealand Journal of Psychiatry*, 32 (5): 698–706.

Hare, E. (1983) 'Was insanity on the increase? The fifty-sixth Maudsley Lecture'. *British Journal of Psychiatry*, 142: 439–55.

Hart, J.T. (1971) 'The inverse care law'. *Lancet*, I: 405–12.

Hartog, J. and Oosterbeek, O. (1998) 'Health, wealth and happiness: why pursue a higher education?' *Economics of Education Review*, 17 (3): 245–56.

Heinrich, J., Popescu, M.A., Wist, M., Goldstein, I.F. and Winchmann, H.E.

(1998) 'Atopy in children and parental social class'. *American Journal of Public Health*, 88 (9): 1319–24.

Hemingway, H., Shipley, M., Macfarlane, P. and Marmot, M. (2000). 'Impact of socioeconomic status on coronary mortality in people with symptoms, electrocardiographic abnormalities, both or neither: the original Whitehall study 25 year follow up'. *Journal of Epidemiology and Community Health*, 54: 510–16.

Heok, K.E., Meng, K.S., Calvin, F.S.L. and Li, T.S. (1996) 'Comorbidity of depression in the elderly: an epidemiological study in a Chinese community'. *International Journal of Geriatric Psychiatry*, 11 (8): 699–704.

Howard, S., Dryden, J. and Johnson, B. (1999) 'Childhood resilience: review and critique of literature'. *Oxford Review of Education*, 25 (3): 307–23.

Hull, B. (1998) 'Education for psychological health'. *Adult Learning*, September, 15–17.

Ippolito, P.M. and Mathios, A.D. (1990) 'Information, advertising and health choices – a study of the cereal market'. *RAND Journal of Economics*, 21 (3): 459–80.

Iverson, L. and Klausen, H. (1981) 'The closure of the Nordhavn shipyard'. Copenhagen: Institute of Social Medicine. Kobenhavns Universitet Publikation 13 FADL.

Jarvis, P. and Walker, J. (1997) 'When the process becomes the product: Summer Universities for seniors'. *Education and Ageing*, 12: 60–8.

Jiang, G.X., Rasmussen, F. and Wasserman, D. (1999) 'Short stature and poor psychological performance: risk factors for attempted suicide among Swedish male conscripts'. *Acta Psychiatrica Scandinavica*, 100 (6): 433–40.

Johnes, G. (1993) *The Economics of Education*. London: Macmillan.

Jorm, A.F., Rodgers, B., Jacomb, P.A., Christensen, H., Henderson, S. and Korten, A.E. (1999) 'Smoking and mental health: results from a community survey'. *Medical Journal of Australia*, 170 (2): 74–7.

Joseph Rowntree Foundation (1995) *Inquiry into Income and Wealth*. York: Joseph Rowntree Foundation.

Karvonen, S., Rimpela, A.H. and Rimpela, M.I. (1999) 'Social mobility and health related behaviours in young people'. *Journal of Epidemiology and Community Health*, 53 (4): 211–17.

Kasenda, M., Calzavara, L.M., Johnson, I. and Le Blanc, M. (1997) 'Correlates of condom use in the young adult population of Ontario'. *Canadian Journal of Public Health*, 88 (4): 280–5.

Kendler, K.S., Neale, M.C., Sullivan, P., Corey, L.A., Gardner, C.O. and Prescott, C.A. (1999) 'A population-based twin study in women of smoking initiation and nicotine dependence'. *Psychological Medicine*, 29 (2): 299–308.

Kenkel, D.S. (1991) Health behavior, health knowledge, and schooling'. *Journal of Political Economy*, 99: 287–305.

Kickbusch, I. (1990) *A Strategy for Health Promotion*. Copenhagen: WHO Regional Office for Europe.

Kiecolt-Glaser, J.K. and Glaser, R. (1986) 'Psychological influences on immunity'. *Psychosomatics*, 27: 621–24.

Kirmayer, L.J., Malus, M. and Boothroyd, L.J. (1996) 'Suicide attempts among Inuit youth: a community survey of prevalence and risk factors'. *Acta Psychiatrica Scandinavia*, 94 (1): 8–17.

Kirpinar, I., Coskun, I., Caykoylu, A., Anac, S. and Ozer, H. (1999) 'First-case postpartum psychoses in Eastern Turkey: a clinical case and follow-up study'. *Acta Psychiatrica Scandinavica*, 100 (3): 199–204.

Kjelsberg, E. (1999) 'A long-term follow-up study of adolescent psychiatric in-patients. Part IV: Predicators of a non-negative outcome'. *Acta Psychiatrica Scandinavica*, 99 (4): 247–51.

Koberg, C.S., Boss, R.W. and Goodman, E. (1998) 'Factors and outcomes associated with mentoring among health-care professionals'. *Journal of Vocational Behavior*, 53 (1): 58–72.

Kocken, P.L. and Voorham, A.J.J. (1998) 'Effects of a peer-led senior health education program'. *Patient Education and Counseling*, 34 (1): 15–23.

Kohn, M.L., Naoi, A., Schoenach, C., Schooler, C. and Slomzcynski, K.M. (1990) 'Position in the class structure and psychological functioning in the United States, Japan and Poland'. *American Journal of Sociology*, 4: 24–52.

Kohn, M.L. and C. Schooler, in collaboration with J. Miller, K.A. Miller, C. Schoenbach and R. Schoenberg (1983) *Work and Personality: An inquiry into the impact of stratification*. Norwood, NJ: Ablex.

Koivusilta, L.K., Rimpela, A.H. and Rimpela, M.K. (1999) 'Health-related lifestyle in adolescence – origin of social class differences in health?' *Health Education Research*, 14 (3): 339–55.

Krause, J.S., Coker, J., Charlifue, S. and Whiteneck, G.G. (1999) 'Depression and subjective well-being among 97 American Indians with spinal cord injury: a descriptive study'. *Rehabilitation Psychology*, 44 (4): 354–372.

Kubzansky, L.D., Berkman, L.F., Glass, T.A. and Seeman, T.E. (1998) 'Is educational attainment associated with shared determinants of health in the elderly? Findings from the MacArthur studies of successful aging'. *Psychosomatic Medicine*, 60 (5): 578–85.

Kubzansky, L.D., Kawachi, I. and Sparrow, D. (1999) ' Socioeconomic status, hostility, and risk factor clustering in the normative aging study: any help from the concept of allostatic load?' *Annals of Behavioral Medicine*, 21 (4): 330–8.

Kunst, A. and Mackenbach, J. (1994) *Measuring Socioeconomic Inequalities in Health*. Copenhagen: World Health Organization Regional Office for Europe.

Kyngas, H. and Lahdenpera, T. (1999) 'Compliance of patients with hypertension and associated factors'. *Journal of Advanced Nursing*, 29 (4): 832–9.

Lawrie, S. and Pelosi, A. (1995) 'Chronic fatigue syndrome in the community: prevalence and associations'. *British Journal of Psychiatry*, 166: 793–7.

Layard, R. (1999) 'Education versus cash redistribution: the lifetime context'. In *Tackling Inequality*. London: Macmillan.

Leigh, J.P. (1990) 'Schooling and seat-belt use'. *Southern Economic Journal*, 57 (1): 195–207.

Leigh, J.P. and Dhir, R. (1997) 'Schooling and frailty among seniors'. *Economics of Education Review*, 16 (1): 45–57.

McEwen, B.S. (2000) 'Allostasis and allostatic load: implications for neuropsycho-pharmacology', *Neuropsychopharmacology*, 22 (2): 108–24.

McGivney, V. (1997), 'Evaluation of the Gloucester Primary Health Care Project'. *GLOSCAT*, unpublished report.

McGivney, V. (2001) 'Fixing or changing the pattern? Reflections on widening adult participation in learning'. Leicester: NIACE.

Mackenbach, J.P. (1993) 'Inequalities in health in the Netherlands according to age, gender, marital status, level of education, degree of organisation, and region'. *European Journal of Public Health*, 3 (2): 112–18.

Mackenbach, J.P., Looman, C.W.N. and Van der Meer, J.B.W. (1996) 'Differences in the misreporting of chronic conditions, by level of education: the effect on inequalities in prevalence rates'. *American Journal of Public Health*, 86 (5): 706–11.

MacLeod, M.C.M., Finlayson, A.R., Pell, J.P., and Findlay, I.N. (1999) 'Geographic, demographic, and socio-economic variations in the investigation and management of coronary heart disease in Scotland'. *British Heart Journal*, 81: 252–6.

McMahon, W. (1999) *Education and Development – Measuring the social benefits*. Oxford: Oxford University Press.

Malmberg, A., Lewis, G., David, A. and Allebeck, P. (1998) 'Premorbid adjustment and personality in people with schizophrenia'. *British Journal of Psychiatry*, 172: 308–13.

Marmot, M.G., Shipley, M.J. and Rose, G. (1984) 'Inequalities in death – specific explanations of a general pattern?' *Lancet*, 1 (8384): 1003–6.

Marmot, M.G., Smith, G.D., Stansfeld, S., Patel, C., North, F., Head, J., White, I., Brunner, E. and Feeney, A. (1991) 'Health inequalities among British civil servants: the Whitehall II study'. *Lancet*, 337 (8754): 1387-93.

Mattiasson, I., Lindgarde, F., Nilsson, J.A., and Therell, T. (1990) 'Threat of unemployment and cardiovascular risk factors: longitudinal study of quality of sleep and serum cholesterol concentrations in men threatened with redundancy'. *British Medical Journal*, 301: 461–6.

Mirowsky, J. and Ross, C.E. (1998) 'Education, personal control, lifestyle and health – a human capital hypothesis'. *Research on Ageing*, 20 (4): 415–49.

Mitchell, R.A., Legge, V. and Sinclair-Legge, G. (1997) 'Membership of the University of the Third Age (U3A) and perceived well-being'. *Disability and Rehabilitation*, 19 (6): 244–8.

Montgomery, S.M. and Schoon, I. (1997) 'Health and health behaviour'. In J. Bynner, E. Ferri and P. Shepherd (eds), *Getting On, Getting By, Getting Nowhere*. Aldershot: Dartmouth.

Mookherjee, H.N. (1998) 'Perception of happiness among elderly persons in metropolitan USA'. *Perceptual and Motor Skills*, 87 (3,1): 787–93.

National Health Strategy (1992) 'Enough to make you sick: how income and environment affect health'. *National Health Strategy Research Paper no. 1*.Canberra, Australia: Department of Health, Housing and Community Services.

Nolan, B. (1990) 'Socioeconomic mortality differentials in Ireland'. *The Economic and Social Review*, 21 (2): 193–208.

Noreau, L., Djon, S.A., Vachon, J., Gervais, M. and Laramee, M.T. (1999) 'Productivity outcomes of individuals with spinal cord injury'. *Spinal Cord*, 37 (10): 730–6.

Ogden, J. (1997) *Health Psychology: A textbook*. Buckingham: Open University Press.

O'Toole, B.I. and Cantor, C. (1995) 'Suicide risk factors among Australian Vietnam era draftees'. *Suicide Life Threat Behavior*, 25 (4): 475–88.

Pappas, G.S., Queen, S., Hadden, W. and Fisher, G. (1993) 'The increasing disparity in mortality between socioeconomic groups in the United States, 1960 and 1986'. *New England Journal of Medicine*, 329: 103–8.

Parry, G., Moyser, G. and Day, N. (1992) *Political Participation and Democracy in Britain*. Cambridge: Cambridge University Press.

Parsons, S. and Bynner, J. (1998) *Influences on Adult Basic Skills*. London: Basic Skills Agency.

Payne, N. and Saul, C. (1997) 'Variations in use of cardiology services in a health authority: comparison of coronary artery revascularisation rates with prevalence of angina and coronary mortality'. *British Medical Journal*, 314: 257–61.

Pearlin, L.I., Lieberman, M.A., Menaghan, E.G. and Mullan, J.T. (1981) 'The stress process'. *Journal of Health and Social Behavior*, 22: 337–56.

Pell, J.P., Pell, A.C.H., Norrie, J., Ford, I. and Cobbe, S.M. (2000) 'Effect of socio-economic deprivation on waiting time for cardiac surgery: retrospective cohort study'. *British Medical Journal*, 320: 15–19.

Perri, T.J. (1984) 'Health status and schooling decisions of young men.' *Economics of Education Review*, 3: 207–13.

Peyrot, M., McMurry, J.F. and Kruger, D.F. (1999) 'A biopsychosocial model of glycemic control in diabetes: stress, coping and regimen adherence'. *Journal of Health and Social Behavior*, 40 (2) 141–58.

Piperno, A. and Di Orio, F. (1990) 'Social differences in health and utilisation of health services in Italy'. In R. Illsley and P.G. Svensson, P.G. (eds), *Social Science and Medicine: Health Inequalities in Europe, Special Issue*, 31 (3): 223–420.

Potter, L.B., Rogler, L.H., Moscicki, E.K. (1995) 'Depression among Puerto Ricans in New York City: the hispanic health and nutrition examination survey'. *Social Psychiatry Psychiatric Epidemiology*, 30 (4): 185–93.

Power, C. and Bartley, M. (1993) 'Health and health service use: sex differences'. In E. Ferri (ed.), *Life at 33: The Fifth Follow-up of the National Child Development Study*. London: National Children's Bureau and City University.

Preston, J. and Hammond, C. (2002) 'The wider benefits of further education: practitioner views'. Wider Benefits of learning Research Report No. 1. London: Centre for Research on the Wider Benefits of Learning, Institute of Education.

Provaznikova, H., Stullerova, N., Stuller, J. and Berkovicova V. (1997) 'Lifestyle, health and achievements of students of the Faculty of Medicine'. *Ceskoslovenska Psychologie*, 41 (3): 216–24.

Psacharopoulos, G. (1994) *Returns to Investment in Education: A global update*. Washington, DC: World Bank.

Putnam, R.D. (1993) *Making Democracy Work: Civic traditions in modern Italy*. Princeton, NJ: Princeton University Press.

Putnam, R.D. (2000) *Bowling Alone: The collapse and revival of American community*. New York: Simon and Schuster.

Resnicow, K., Smith, M., Harrison, L. and, Drucker, E. (1999) 'Correlates of occasional cigarette and marijuana use: are teens harm reducing?' *Addictive Behaviors*, 24 (2): 251–66.

Richards, H., McConnachie, A., Morrison, C., Murray, K. and Watt, G. (2000) 'Social and gender variation in the prevalence, presentation and general practitioner provisional diagnosis of chest pain'. *Journal of Epidemiology and Community Health*, 54: 714–18.

Rini, C.K., DunkelSchetter, C., Wadhwa, P.D. and Sandman, C.A. (1999) 'Psychological adaptation and birth outcomes: the role of personal resources, stress, and sociocultural context in pregnancy'. *Health Psychology*, 18 (4): 333–45.

Rodriguez-Garcia, T. and Goldman, P. (1994) *The Health Development Link*. Washington, DC: Pan American Health Organization/ WHO.

Rose, M.J. (2000) *Future Tense. Are the growing occupations more stressed-out and depressive?* Working Paper 5, ESRC Future of Work Programme. Swindon: ESRC.

Rosenweig, M.R. and Schultz, T.P. (1981) 'Education and household production of child health.' In *Proceedings of the American Statistical Association (Social Statistics Section)*, Washington, DC: American Statistical Association: 53–92.

Ross, C.E. and Mirowsky, J. (1999) 'Refining the association between education and health: the effects of quantity, credential, and selectivity.' *Demography*, 36 (4): 445–60.

Rudman, L.A., Gonzales, M.H. and Borgida, E. (1999) 'Mishandling the gift of life: Noncompliance in renal transplant patients'. *Journal of Applied Social Psychology*, 29 (4): 834–51.

Rutter, M. (1990) 'Psychosocial resilience and protective mechanisms'. In J. Rolf, A. Masten, D. Cicchetti, K. Neuchterlein, and S. Weintraub (eds) *Risk and Protective Factors in the Development of Psychopathology*, New York: Cambridge University Press.

Sander, W. (1995a) 'Schooling and quitting smoking'. *Review of Economics and Statistics*, 77: 191–9.

Sander, W. (1995b) 'Schooling and smoking'. *Economics of Education Review*, 14: 23–33.

Schafer, E., Schafer, R.B., Keith, P.M. and Bose, J. (1999) 'Self-esteem and fruit and vegetable intake in women and men'. *Journal of Nutrition Education*, 31 (3): 153–60.

Seeman, M. and Lewis, S. (1995) 'Powerlessness, health and mortality: a longitudinal study of older men and mature women'. *Social Science and Medicine*, 41: 517–25.

Seeman, M. and Seeman, T.E. (1983) 'Health behavior and personal autonomy: a longitudinal study of older men and mature women'. *Social Science and Medicine*, 41: 517–25.

Seeman, M., Seeman, A.Z. and Budros, A. (1988) 'Powerlessness, work and community: a longitudinal study of alienation and alcohol use'. *Journal of Health and Social Behavior*, 29: 185–98.

Shakotko, R.A., Edwards, L.N. and Grossman, M. (1981). 'An exploration of the dynamic relationship between health and cognitive development in adolescence'. In J. van der Gaag and M. Perlman (eds) *Contributions to Economic Analysis: Health, economics, and health economics*. Amsterdam: North-Holland Publishing Company.

Shefer, A., Dobbins, J. and Fukuda, K. (1997) 'Fatiguing illness among employees in three large state office buildings, California, 1993: was there an outbreak?' *Journal of Psychosomatic Research*, 31: 31–43.

Sihvonen, A.P., Kunst, A.E., Lahelma, E., Valkonen, T. and Mackenbach, J.P. (1998) 'Socioeconomic inequalities in health expectancy in Finland and Norway in the late 1980s'. *Social Science and Medicine*, 47 (3): 303–15.

Slater, M.D., Basil, M.D. and Mailbach, E.W. (1999) 'A cluster analysis of alcohol-related attitudes and behaviours in the general population'. *Journal of Studies on Alcohol*, 60 (5): 667–74.

Sloggett, A. and Joshi, H. (1998) 'Deprivation indicators as predictors of life events, 1981–1992, based on the UK ONS longitudinal study'. *Journal of Epidemiology and Community Health*, 52 (4): 228–33.

Stevens, F.C.J., Kaplan, C.D., Ponds, R.W.H.M., Diederiks, J.P.M. and Jolles, J. (1999) 'How ageing and social factors affect memory.' *Age and Ageing*, 28 (4): 379–84.

Taubman, P. and Rosen, S. (1982) 'Healthiness, education, and marital status.'

In V.R. Fuchs (ed.) *Economic Aspects of Health*. Chicago: University of Chicago Press for the National Bureau of Economic Research.

Teisl, M.F., Lew, A.S. and Derby, B.M. (1999) 'The effects of education and information source on consumer awareness of diet-disease relationships'. *Journal of Public Policy and Marketing*, 18 (2): 197–207.

Thompson, R.L., Margetts, B.M., Speller, V.M. and McVey, D. (1999) 'The Health Education Authority's health and lifestyle survey 1993: who are the low fruit and vegetable consumers?' *Journal of Epidemiology and Community Health*, 53 (5): 294–9.

Toppelberg, C.O. and Shapiro, T. (2000) 'Language disorders: a 10-year research update review'. *Journal of the American Academy of Child and Adolescent Psychiatry*, 39 (2): 143–52.

Toro, K., Nicolau, R., Cervera, M., Castro, J., Blecua, M.J., Zaragoza, M. and Toro, A. (1995) 'A clinical and phenomenological study of 185 Spanish adolescents with anorexia-nervosa'. *European Child and Adolescent Psychiatry*, 4 (3): 165–74.

Turk, D.C., Meichenbaum, D. and Genest, M. (1983) *Pain and Behavioural Medicine*. New York: Guildford Press.

Turner, J.B. (1995). 'Economic context and the effects of unemployment'. *Journal of Health and Social Behaviour*, 213: 36–229.

Turner, H.A. and Turner, R.J. (1999) 'Gender, social status, and emotional reliance'. *Journal of Health and Social Behavior*, 40 (4): 360–73.

Uchino, B.N., Cacioppo, J.T., and Kiecolt-Glaser, J.K. (1996) 'The relationship between social support and physiological processes: a review with emphasis on underlying mechanisms and implications for health'. *Psychological Bulletin*, 119 (3): 488–531.

Ullah, P. (1990) 'The association between income, financial strain and psychological well-being among unemployed youths'. *Journal of Occupational Psychology*, 63: 317–30.

Vagero, D. and Lundberg, O. (1989) 'Health inequalities in Britain and Sweden'. *The Lancet*, ii: 35–6.

Valkonen, T. (1993) 'Problems in the measurement and international comparisons of socioeconomic differences in mortality'. *Social Science and Medicine*, 36 (4): 409–18.

Van Oers, J.A.M., Bongers, I.M.B., Van de Goor, L.A.M. and Garretsen, H.F.L. (1999) 'Alcohol consumption, alcohol-related problems, problem drinking, and socio-economic status'. *Alcohol and Alcoholism*, 34 (1): 78–88.

Varenna, M., Binelli, I., Zucchi, F., Ghiringhelli, D., Gallazzi, M. and Sinigaglia, L. (1999) 'Prevalence of osteoporosis by educational level in a cohort of postmenopausal women'. *Osteoporosis International*, 9 (3): 236–41.

Veenhoven, R. (1996) 'Developments in satisfaction research'. *Social Indicators Research*, 37: 1–46.

Veenstra, G. (2000) 'Social capital, SES and health: and individual-level analysis.' *Social Science and Medicine*, 50 (5): 619–29.

Vega Dienstmaier, J.M., Mazzotti, G., Stucchi Portocarrero, S. and Campos, M. (1999) 'Prevalence and risk factors for depression in postpartum women'. *Actas espanolas de psiquiatria*, 27 (5): 299–303.

Viramo, P., Luukinen, H., Koski, K., Laippala, P., Sulkava, R. and Kivela, S.L. (1999)'Orthostatic hypotension and cognitive decline in older people'. *Journal of the American Geriatrics Society*, 47 (5): 600–4.

Wadsworth, M.E.J. (1997) 'Changing social factors and their long-term implications for health'. *British Medical Bulletin*, 53 (1): 198–209.

Wagner, U. and Zick, A. (1995) 'The relation of formal education to ethnic prejudice: its reliability, validity and explanation'. *European Journal of Social Psychology*, 25 (1): 41–56.

Wagstaff, A. (1986) 'The demand for health: some new empirical evidence'. *Journal of Health Economics*, 5: 195–233.

Wamala, S.P., Mittleman, M.A., Schenck Gustafsson, K. and Orth Gomer, K. (1999) 'Potential explanations for the educational gradient in coronary heart disease: a population-based case-control study of Swedish women'. *American Journal of Public Health*, 89 (5): 785.

Wang, M.C. (1997) 'Next steps in inner-city education: focusing on reliance, development and learning success'. *Education and Urban Society*, 29 (3): 255–76.

Weilgos, C.M. and Cunningham, W.R. (1999) 'Age-related slowing on the digit symbol task: longitudinal and cross-sectional analyses'. *Experimental Aging Research*, 99 (25): 109–20.

Wertheimer, A. (1997) *Images of Possibility. Creating learning opportunities for adults with mental health difficulties*. Leicester: National Institute of Adult Continuing Education.

Wessely, S., Hotoph, M. and Sharpe, M. (1998). *Chronic fatigue and its syndromes*. Oxford: Oxford University Press.

West, L. (1995) 'Beyond fragments: adults, motivation and higher education'. *Studies in the Education of Adults*, 27 (2): 133–56.

Westermeyer, J. and Specker, S. (1999) 'Social resources and social function in comorbid eating and substance disorder: a matched pairs study'. *American Journal on Addictions*, 8 (4): 332–6.

Wheaton, B. (1980) 'The sociogenesis of psychological disorder: an attributional theory'. *Journal of Health and Social Behavior*, 21: 100–24.

Wheeler, M., Smith, F., and Trayhorn, L. (1999) *Improving Health through Referral to Adult Education*. Report produced by the Kingston and Richmond Health Authority and the Royal Borough of Kingston-upon-Thames.

Whelan, C.T. (1991) 'The role of income, life-style deprivation and financial strain in mediating the impact of unemployment on psychological distress: evidence from the Republic of Ireland'. Unpublished mimeograph from The Economic and Social Research Institute, Dublin.

Whitty, G., Aggleton, P., Gamarnikow, E. and Tyrer, P. (1998) 'Independent inquiry into inequalities in health: Input paper 10 to the Independent Inquiry into Inequalities in Health'. *Journal of Education Policy*, 13 (5): 641–52.

Wilkinson, R.G. (1996) *Unhealthy Societies: The afflictions of inequality*. London: Routledge.

Wittchen, H.U., Fuetsch, M., Sonntag, H., Muller, N. and Liebowitz M (1999) 'Disability and quality of life in pure and comorbid social phobia – findings from a controlled study'. *European Psychiatry*, 14 (3): 118–31.

Wittchen, H.U., Nelson, C.B. and Lachner, G. (1998) 'Prevalence of mental disorders and psychosocial impairments in adolescents and young adults'. *Psychological Medicine*, 28 (1): 109–26.

Wolfe, B.L. (1985) 'The influence of health on school outcomes: a multivariate approach'. *Medical Care*, 23: 1127–38.

Wolinsky, F.D., Wyrwich, K.W., Jung, S.C. and Gurney, J.G. (1999) 'The risk of hospitalisation for acute myocardial infarction among older adults'. *Journals of Gerontology Series A – Biological Sciences and Medical Sciences*, 54 (5): M254–M261.

World Bank (1993) *World Bank Development Report*. New York: World Bank.

World Bank (1994) *Uganda: Social Sectors: A World Bank Country Study*. New York: World Bank.

Wottiez, I. and Theuwes, J. (1998) 'Well-being and labor market status'. In S.P. Jenkins, A. Kapteyn and B. Van Praag (eds), *The Distribution of Welfare and Household Production*: 211–32.